The Document Method

IØØ49224

Programs of Projects to Optimize Healthcare

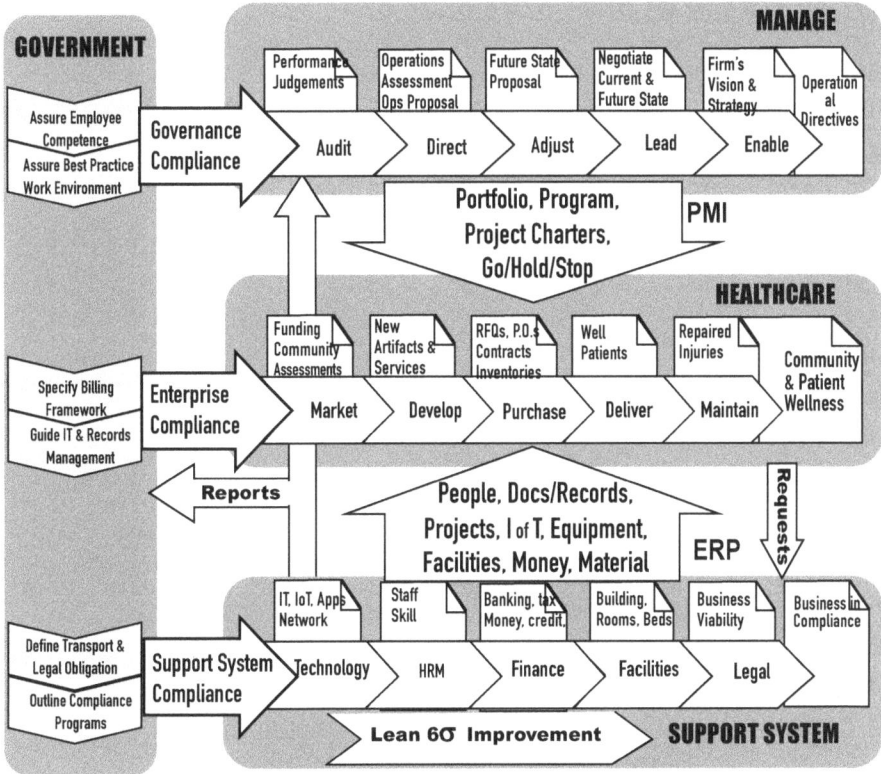

Healthcare System Models

Jim I. Jones

3rd edition: Copyright © 2020 by Jim I. Jones
2nd edition: Copyright © 2007 by Jim I. Jones
1st edition: Copyright © 1999 by Jim I. Jones

Printed in the United States of America

ISBN: 978-0-9672159-3-8

LCCN: 2025901366

Author / Publisher: Jim I. Jones

Dewey Decimal Classification
DDC: 610.285 - Medical Informatics
Keywords: Artificial intelligence, machine learning, healthcare informatics, patient data systems, medical technology.

DDC: 362.1068 - Healthcare Quality Improvement and Process Optimization
Keywords: Process optimization, resource management, Lean Six Sigma, healthcare administration, quality improvement.

Healthcare costs have reached staggering proportions, consuming 17.5% of GDP in the U.S. and 11% in the EU. This upward trajectory is alarming and financially unsustainable.

Albert Einstein once said, "I want to know God's thoughts; the rest are details." While I lack Einstein's insight, addressing these issues requires meticulous attention to detail. This need for precision inspired the creation of The Document Methodology (TDM), originally developed in manufacturing over 20 years ago. Since the first publication of TDM in 1999, its principles have been applied across diverse industries, with subsequent updates in 2007, 2020, and now a portfolio in 2025.

This Portfolio defines programs to combat the rising costs of healthcare while enhancing patient wellness. Using TDM, it outlines a portfolio of programs and projects designed to improve patient flow, optimize resource utilization, and reduce expenses. This endeavor is complex but essential to achieving better healthcare outcomes at a lower cost. Project 5.6 in Chapter 6 provides insight to continuously improve operations everywhere in a hospital by leveraging neural network and discrete event simulations.

Why Documents?

Documents, in their many forms—from ancient carvings to digital records—have always been the cornerstone of knowledge preservation and process management. TDM leverages this 6,000-year legacy, integrating static and dynamic models to measure, manage, and improve processes. It depends on advanced document management systems, workflow tools, Health Information Systems (HIS), artificial intelligence (AI), and robust IT infrastructure.

TDM's Evolution

Many readers may be seasoned professionals with deep tacit knowledge in engineering, medicine, or other fields. This book bridges the gap between specialized expertise and the underlying principles of process improvement. Drawing from my experience in manufacturing, TDM III contrasts industrial practices with healthcare systems. Given that U.S. healthcare costs have skyrocketed from $27.2 billion in 1960 ($290 billion in today's dollars) to $4800 billion in 2023, there is an urgent need for innovative approaches, particularly for elder care. Effective care for seniors must prioritize quality of life and well-being over prolonging life at any cost. For example, in-home paramedicine supported by telemedicine can often provide better outcomes for frail seniors than emergency room visits.

Systems Engineering in Healthcare

From a systems engineering perspective, patients are complex, adaptive systems requiring tailored portfolios of diagnosis, treatment, and rehabilitation projects. These structured value streams ensure comprehensive care while optimizing resource utilization. The book's graphical models reveal the intricacies of medical diagnosis, treatment workflows, and process improvements, making TDM a uniquely comprehensive tool for healthcare reform.

The Community Impact

Improving healthcare is not just about individual well-being; it's about strengthening the fabric of communities. By enhancing senior care and addressing healthcare inefficiencies, we can reduce costs while improving quality of life. This collaborative approach fosters a sense of shared responsibility and mutual support within communities.

Throughout this book, you will find process diagrams illustrating various workflows. These visual aids provide clarity, linking tasks, outputs, and supporting technologies. The appendices include a sample record retention schedule, a draft healthcare delivery model, a proposal for healthcare reform in the U.S. and an IEEE submission on Ethics in Engineering.

Acknowledgements are on the last page, but I owe a special thanks to Judith G. Jones (BA, RN, WIFE) for her invaluable contributions to all four editions of this work. Her efforts were especially valuable because she is a registered nurse that can spell.

By embracing TDM, we can create a sustainable, efficient, and patient-centric healthcare system. It is my hope that this book inspires readers to take on the challenge and contribute to this vital mission. For those who take on the challenge, review the projects, especially those in Chapter 6.

jimijones@aol.com

This book details an extensive framework, The Document Methodology (TDM), designed to optimize healthcare systems by focusing on knowledge management, process optimization, and technology integration. The methodology, originally applied to manufacturing, addresses the pressing issues of unsustainable healthcare costs and improving patient outcomes and operational efficiency.

Central to TDM "documents as knowledge flow," recognize documents as crucial vehicles for transforming raw data into actionable insights. Documents are categorized into five types: Knowledge, Transaction, Management, Capability, and External, each critical to healthcare delivery.

TDM emphasizes the importance of creating a structured taxonomy for critical documents to facilitate efficient knowledge retrieval and utilization. This taxonomy aligns with ISO 15489 standards, ensuring document authenticity, reliability, integrity, and usability.

TDM leverages portfolio management to organize and manage healthcare initiatives. This approach facilitates a holistic view of the healthcare system, enabling strategic planning, resource allocation, and performance monitoring across all levels. Key aspects of the portfolio approach include:

- Patient-Centric Portfolios: Each patient is considered a project in the portfolio, dedicated to the patient's flow to wellness.
- Project Focus: Designed to address specific health areas (e.g., diabetes mitigation, cardiac health) focused on tailored interventions.
- Managing Projects in Portfolios: Doctors and healthcare systems can manage a portfolio of patients, enabling efficient resource allocation.

TDM also emphasizes the integration of advanced technologies:

- Health IT and ERP Systems are leveraged for effective data management and analysis.
- Artificial Intelligence (AI) is integrated to optimize clinical decision support and resource utilization.
- Internet of Things (IoT) and RFIDs facilitate real-time adjustments and improvements in healthcare operations.

The portfolio outlines five programs to drive healthcare transformation:

- Program 1: Facilitate Healthcare with Knowledge and Technology.
- Program 2: Optimize Process by Modelling Healthcare Systems.
- Program 3: Empower Employees to Effectively Deliver Healthcare.
- Program 4: Enhance Support Systems for Healthcare.

- Program 5: Optimize Patient Flow to Wellness.

Lean Six Sigma principles are integrated throughout TDM, ensuring continuous process improvement and data-driven decision-making. The framework highlights the use of Lean Value Stream Mapping for patient flow analysis and the application of discrete event simulations to optimize resource allocation and reduce wait times.

TDM extends beyond the traditional healthcare setting by incorporating the concept of community and patient wellness. It recognizes the importance of addressing social determinants of health and advocates for community engagement, health education, and preventative care initiatives.

The implementation of TDM requires a structured approach that involves:
- Executive Assessment: A preliminary review of content-related issues, potential solutions, and business benefits.
- Document Strategy, Policy Report and Proposal: Identifies content-related processes, systems, and initiatives, major issues and solutions.
- Specification for Process Innovation: Maps, analyzes, and benchmarks business process to identify inefficiencies and propose improvements.
- Knowledge and Work Practice Assessment: Creates a basis for managing knowledge flow, cultural practices, and social capital, proposing a plan for business transformation.
- Solution Requirements Specification: Defines business and technical requirements for a service.
- Business Case: Develops a cost-benefit justification for a project.

TDM provides a comprehensive roadmap for transforming healthcare systems, emphasizing knowledge management, process optimization, technology integration, and a patient-centric approach. This framework holds the potential to address the growing challenges of healthcare costs, improve patient outcomes, and create a more sustainable and efficient healthcare ecosystem. Key areas for further development include:
- Developing detailed Python simulations: While the document outlines the conceptual framework to simulate patient flow and resource allocation, more work is needed to implement the Python code.
- Integrating TDM into existing Health IT and ERP systems: The success of TDM depends on seamless integration with healthcare data systems.
- Collecting and managing high-quality data: The effectiveness of AI and simulation models relies on ISO15489 compliant healthcare records.

TABLE OF CONTENTS

Table of Contents

Table of Figures

PORTFOLIO

Portfolio Background

This portfolio defines programs and projects for anyone trying to manage, operate, understand a medical complex, which is supported by an information system on a computer network and Internet of Things (IoT).

Fact-based management is rare except in manufacturing where process is explicitly defined, and flow-to-value is monitored: components flow through fabrication to create product value. Evidence based medicine notwithstanding, patient flow to wellness is not easy to explicitly define.

The Document Methodology (TDM) asserts that the ability to compete on knowledge is dependent upon any enterprise's ability to explicitly define, monitor and continuously improve knowledge flow-to-value for products and (patient) services.

A document may contain noise, data, information or knowledge. Noise is an incomprehensible jumble of images and text. Data can result from monitoring events or is derived from other data. Information is the result of summarizing or correlating data; it is data organized into patterns and visualized to create insights that support decisions. Knowledge is actionable information because it has meaning (in recorded and unrecorded form); it has been validated from collaboration, and quality of method; analytical, statistical and logical methods are used to build an information base that is reviewed by a peer group to validate structure and content.

Figure: 1-1 illustrates the transition from noise to knowledge flow to value. Value in manufacturing is primarily driven by competition in the marketplace and as such can be determined from many forms of market analysis and statistics where customers know the price of products.

NOISE	DATA	INFORMATION	KNOWLEDGE
INCOMPREHENSIBLE IMAGES AND SOUNDS	UNORGANIZED NUMBERS, WORDS, SOUNDS, IMAGES	DATA ARRANGED AND PROCESSED INTO MEANINGFUL CONTENT	CONTENT VALIDATED FOR PRODUCTIVE USE, MADE ACTIONABLE

NOISE, DATA, CONTENT OR KNOWLEDGE
STRUCTURED & PUBLISHED FOR PEOPLE

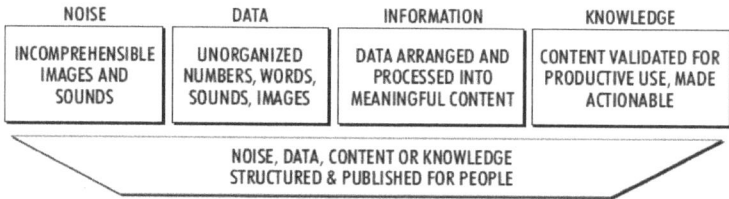

Figure 1-1: Document

Modern economists subscribe to the *Subjective Theory of Value*: economic value comes not from any quality of the good in question, but from the human mind. Paradoxically, in healthcare prices aren't even listed for patients to see. Many people who have insurance think it's free and indulge in tests and diagnoses that aren't indicated by their malady or opt for an intervention that they would not opt for if they had to pay for it. To compound this problem, healthy people devalue insurance until they require major medical attention at which point they want to purchase insurance. This is not the dynamics of Adam Smith's capitalism.

TDM taxonomy uses library science classification that contains a full set of entries for all key organizational documents identified by process models in knowledge flow to value. It is critical that a taxonomy uniquely identifies key documents with metadata that support knowledge flow to value. These models inform management how to define policy, goals, objectives and a portfolio of programs for its transformation.

The Document Methodology

Chapters 2-6 are devoted to each of the topics below. This introductory chapter provides an overview of the details in the diagram. When The Document Methodology (TDM) is fully applied, the resources and technology available to an enterprise can optimize healthcare operations and accelerate the flow of patients to wellness. It is based on:

Knowledge of the enterprise (hospital system), found in documents.

Processes that define hospital operation and depend on documents for definition, initiation and tracking.

People who use facts from documents and patient monitored data and have the skills to manage and change processes.

Systems that provide capabilities to manage and improve operations.

Operations that are facilitated by documents, AI, simulation and HIT.

To manage knowledge within an enterprise, the enterprise's body of knowledge must be identified and defined. Knowledge includes cognition, skills, theories, rules, processes, techniques, instructions for action used by the enterprise to solve problems and to produce output (patient outcomes), some of which have been recorded in documents and some of which is unrecorded. A document is paper, electronic, optical or some other form of technology. Other knowledge resides in the minds and skills of staff.

Knowledge is captured in a variety of ways. Specialists collaborate to explicitly capture knowledge in documents based on their tacit knowledge and skills. Other knowledge is created and put into documents (and records) that can be productively described by business cases. However, knowledge must also be catalogued (such as with key words) and stored in ways that can be found with sophisticated searches.

Once a body of knowledge is defined, knowledge objects are derived which are critical knowledge used by a firm to produce value for its customers; examples include information recorded in documents (i.e., patient electronic health records), core competency in staff (i.e., specialist skills or diagnostician), and information embedded in facilities, equipment and processes (i.e., laboratory, operating theater, ER procedures).

Once identified, a set of measurable enterprise processes and value-added outputs which utilize the knowledge objects can be defined. Examples of output having value can be products, a document, an approval, diagnosis, surgery, drug therapy, etc. The knowledge objects are used in monitored processes in order to measure the knowledge flow to value (the time it takes the knowledge object to flow through the process to create the output). From this point of view, a patient becomes a repository (recorded in an EHR) of medical staff knowledge and skills as s/he flows through a medical process that may or may not result in a positive outcome (i.e., cured of cancer). The enterprise processes can then be modified using a continuous improvement framework repeatedly to optimize knowledge flow to value.

Documents are an explicit form of enterprise communication and contain data, information and knowledge formatted for people. All explicit communication between people is a document: written, oral, electronic, paper, video, audio or physical prototype. This definition of documents subordinates them to data, information and knowledge. Repositories are "libraries" of documents: physical or electronic.

In healthcare, patients' EHR as well as the documented symptom/cause diagnoses of physicians' intervention-rehabilitation plans contain value-added knowledge to produce positive patient outcomes. This knowledge is built into technology, work instruction documents and the core competencies of the enterprise's staff. Potential value is built into the development process, where people create new products or better patient services and record their specific attributes in R&D documents for better products/outcomes in the future. The cost and rate at which value is added or created has a significant effect on an organization's wealth.

Also, the skills of a paramedic collaborating via a telemedicine link with an ER physician can save a life. This knowledge is built into technology, work instruction documents and core competencies of people.

Models for The Document Methodology

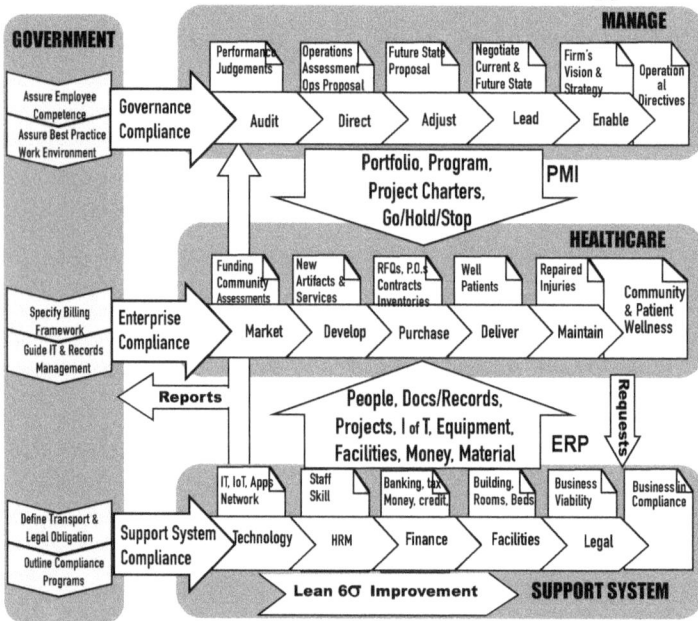

Figure 1-2: *Healthcare System Models*

The document describes a comprehensive, integrated model for managing healthcare systems illustrated if Figure 1-2, specifically focused on patient flow from admission to discharge, using Lean and Value Stream Mapping techniques. It is structured to optimize allocation of resources such as medical staff, equipment, and facilities across various hospital zones. The model integrates government, management, healthcare, and support systems to achieve patient and community wellness, emphasizing continuous communication and adaptive management.

Key Context Models

Government model assumes that it knows how to regulate a capitalistic society which is clearly not true. The World Economic Federation rates the USA 30th or below in its four basic pillars upon which it evaluates countries' basic business environments. Overall, the USA rates 2nd only to Singapore as a place to do business, so government blundering hasn't kept business from being successful. However, government's 629 healthcare regulations raise cost and potentially reduce quality of care.

Manage model represents every person (not just senior managers) in the organization. This model continuously communicates with the Healthcare Model via a "Portfolio, Program, Project Charter" structure which is continuously revised in the "Audit" function resulting in a, Go/Hold/Stop directive on instantiated programs or projects. Management is directing someone including oneself in tasks that work toward improving the service (patient wellness) or corporate viability (sustainable profitability). Management task result in a "Directive" (not a service or product). Its output can be framed by a portfolio of programs and project charters to direct an activity. This could be >100 pages or a half page for an individual.

Healthcare model improves patient and community health and generate payrolls and profit. However, the capitalistic profit motive, keeps USA healthcare at a cost that is higher than anywhere else in the world.

System Support model is the mechanism that assures the efficient, effective, adaptive operation of the Healthcare model. It supplies, maintains, and improves "People, Records, Projects, IoT, Equipment, Facilities, Money, Material," communications, networks, infrastructure, information, history, contracts, compliance, and relationships.

Key Processes

- Patient Care Flow: Emphasizes Michael Porter's Integrated Practice Unit (IPU) model, focusing on coordinated, multidisciplinary care based on specific medical conditions. The approach is adapted to address delays and waiting times, which constitute the majority of patient experience while awaiting critical resources or services.
- Lean Value Stream Mapping: Models patient flow as a series of zones with critical and ubiquitous care areas. By mapping out bottlenecks and wait times, the model aims to predict resource usage for a 5-day horizon, adjusting for patient priorities and resource availability.
- **iDEF0** provides a unique approach to showing the FLOW of knowledge making it an effective tool for SEEING business anomalies. To frame a simulation, process hierarchies must be viable.

Data and Systems Integration

- Patient Data Capture: Comprehensive data, including demographics, medical history, and treatment details, is managed to ensure patient safety and streamline transitions across hospital zones.
- Health Information Technology (HIT): Systems like EPIC or Cerner are used to schedule and track entities to support patient flow to wellness.
- Neural Network Simulation: Diagnose patient wellness from symptoms.
- Discrete Event Simulation: Simulate and track patient flow to wellness.
- Value Stream Analysis and Lean 6σ predict and optimize outcomes.

Typical Patient Flows (Value Streams)

- Standardized Value Streams for Medicare DRGs (Diagnostic-Related-Group: e.g., joint replacement, sepsis, heart failure) define the patient journey from initiation, diagnosis, intervention, custodial care, rehabilitation, discharge, to post-discharge follow-up.

Critical Resources

- Job Classes: Defined roles for physicians, nurses, specialists, and other support staff who interact at various points in patient care.
- Facilities and Equipment: MRI machines, ICU beds, operating rooms, and support facilities, critical for maintaining patient flow.

- Laboratories and Therapies: Clinical support units (e.g., labs for diagnostics, physical therapy) are outlined as crucial for patient assessment and recovery.

Lean Six Sigma

Lean Six Sigma uses operational data to determine how to change the hospital to a more effective, efficient higher quality future state by defining Rapid Improvement Events (RIE: just do it, do it now, do it fast) to take baby steps in the right direction.

Summary: The top-down model for the healthcare system plus the Care Model with a patient Value Stream Map using patient RFIDs, leads to a Discrete Event Simulation (DES) that continuously monitors a portfolio of patient projects that flow through critical scheduled areas of the hospital as well as time spent waiting. This will require a Portfolio manager who oversees flow to adjust staff, resource and facility assignments in real time.

Five Axioms of The Document Methodology

The Document Methodology is founded on five core axioms, each underscoring the pivotal role of documents in shaping and improving enterprise operations, particularly in healthcare. These axioms guide how organizations manage knowledge, processes, and change effectively.

Axiom 1: Documents Record Enterprise Knowledge

Documents represent an organization's collective knowledge. They encapsulate insights, interpretations, analyses, and systems in forms such as text, graphics, videos, and other media. The types of documents include:
- Knowledge Documents: Specialized insights that drive patient wellness.
- Transaction Documents: Initiate and record process activities.
- Management Documents: Strategic directions and operational facts.
- Capability Documents: Outline enterprise capacities and availability.
- External Documents: Address regulations within which a firm operates.

Axiom 2: Documents Define Enterprise Processes

Every value-added step within an enterprise relies on documentation. Processes are either driven by documents, altered through documentation, or replicated using documents for initiation. Documents provide the foundation for analyzing and improving business operations by:

- Driving Processes: Lack of documentation can cause bottlenecks. Improving document flow and content accelerates processes.
- Defining Processes: The flow of documents provides a clear lens through which business operations can be understood and optimized.

By linking documents to process states, people, and technologies, a firm can create process models that be used to streamline operations and promote continuous improvement.

Axiom 3: Documents Provide Facts to Manage People

Explicitly defined and tracked processes enable managers to access real-time facts about operations. With these facts, managers can:

- Refine process workflows.
- Reallocate resources to address constraints.
- Reduce costs or improve quality.

Documents allow for transparent tracking, enabling empowered employees to self-manage and continuously audit processes for performance improvements. This axiom emphasizes leadership as recognizing what to change and how to implement changes effectively to create value.

Axiom 4: Documents Structure Support Systems

IT and AI support systems rely on documents to provide the knowledge needed for efficient operations. To make enterprise knowledge accessible:

- Documents are categorized with metadata, taxonomy, and keywords.
- Systems must be secure, reliable, searchable information repositories.

Documents form the backbone of support systems, enabling employees to retrieve and utilize the precise knowledge needed to perform their roles effectively. Advanced technologies, including mobile tools and AI, can further enhance the accessibility and usability of documents.

Axiom 5: Documents Guide Enterprise Operations and Change

For any improvement effort, the key question is: "What should change?" Documents play a critical role in answering this question by:

- Recording historical knowledge and actions.
- Providing data necessary to evaluate process variations and bottlenecks.
- Offering the foundation for simulations and planning future changes.

While no enterprise system fully documents all processes due to dynamic factors like human behavior and unforeseen events, a well-documented system significantly improves a firm's ability to adapt and innovate.

The five axioms collectively highlight that documents are far more than static records. They are dynamic tools for preserving knowledge, defining processes, managing operations, supporting systems, and driving change.

Portfolio Introduction

Vision: Model healthcare to pre-qualify capability to deliver integrated, transparent, accountable regional urban and rural healthcare and long-term care sustained by a major hospital.

Discussion

Healthcare and wellness groups collaborate to sustain a "healthy" community. This is guided by the fact that Intermountain Healthcare in Utah has the healthiest population at the lowest per-capita health care costs, according to some measures. Utah's per-capita cost is just over half those of equally healthy Massachusetts ($5,013 vs. $9,278). Brent James, MD, executive director at Intermountain's Institute for Health Care Leadership, says that 60% to 70% of the state's 3 million people identify as Mormon and most of them follow the church's dietary and behavioral restrictions, which include no tobacco, alcohol, or recreational drugs. The faith also encourages large families and strong social networks, both of which provide support when people get sick.

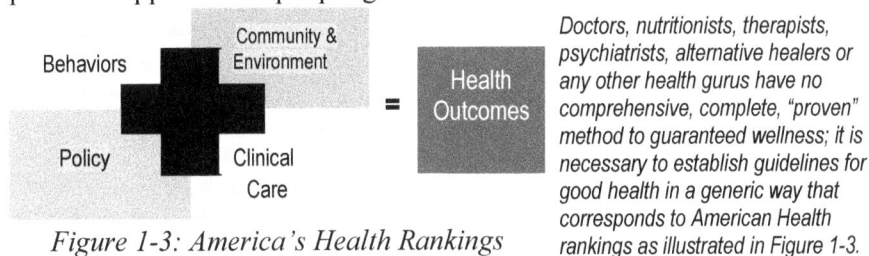

Figure 1-3: America's Health Rankings

Doctors, nutritionists, therapists, psychiatrists, alternative healers or any other health gurus have no comprehensive, complete, "proven" method to guaranteed wellness; it is necessary to establish guidelines for good health in a generic way that corresponds to American Health rankings as illustrated in Figure 1-3.

There must also be a way to validate that some, part, or all of those guidelines are relevant to wellness. The general approach must treat the health system's community as a (but not randomized) clinical trial.

Five Dimensions of the Medical Environment

- Policy provides guidelines and allocates budgets by arbitrating effective and efficient operations with continuous, innovative, adaptive change to improve health outcomes and insure Federal, state and best practice compliance

- Culture makes information meaningful, in terms of interpreting staff's experience and helping them decide how to act.

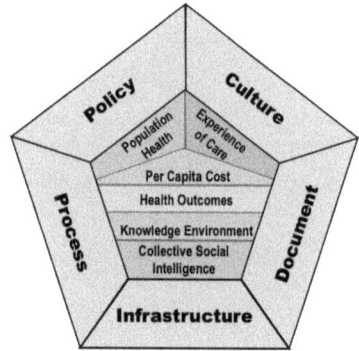

- Document/content is focused on presenting information to invoke desirable behaviors in the information consumer (e.g. medical staff: quicker diagnosis, ER).

- Process represents the tasks that staff perform to create value for the patient. It must support measurement.

- Infrastructure/Architecture using global information networks, collaboration technologies and the web is deployed to support and ensure that knowledge flows to positive experience of care, improved population health and reduced per capita cost.

Drivers

Policy	Culture	Content	Process	Infrastructure
Define an internally billable quality project, as part of a review, to improve, validate, integrate and synchronize Work Instructions and submit them to quality for sign-off & global distribution.	Knowledge sharing Continuous Improvement Formal mentoring Patient offsite consultat Standardized work practices across geography Formal CoPs for IPU groups & peer communications Patient and project centric organization Rewards consistent with sharing & project behavior	Web based documents Electronic SOAP/ OODA submissions EHR validation Patient portfolio history stored in a DMS. Work Instructions, & check sheets synchronized.	WI & changes integral to processes Peer review Work Instruction validation drives changes and streamlines project planning. Project teams	Portal Document Workflow ICM system

To mitigate the consequence of healthcare costs exceeding 17.5% of U.S. GDP, a healthcare system model includes institutions and the community and enumerates possibilities for technology improvement and the ways healthcare is delivered. The model quantifies and qualifies targets for capability development and continuous improvement using technologies for telehealth and telemedicine, and transport facilities and disseminating best practices, R&D and innovation.

Since documents are ubiquitous to every environment associated with wellness and healthcare, a taxonomy of information (documents) must be defined that supports such a view of information; the approach must:

- Educate the community in a language (supported by taxonomy) to communicate symptoms, illness, habits, and history.
- Validate everything that gets recorded in the EHR to assure ISO 15489 compliance.
- Revise the nurse SOAP note framework into a structure that will make it better for analysis by artificial intelligence algorithms.
- Track not only the cost per patient, but the cost to promote wellness with the community.
- Initiate health fairs to communicate healthy behaviors and how to identify symptoms that are indicators of medical problems.
- Define guidelines to ensure wellness, reduce cost of care, minimize patient risk and maximize positive outcomes.
- Install a Clinical Diagnosis System (CDS) to leverage rigorous recording of patient and community data and physician team diagnosis.
- Support the above objectives with information technology and telemedicine wherever possible.

Set of Key Performance Indicators
Critical to judging whether the projects and actions being performed are achieving enterprise goals and objectives is to monitor and report on programs with respect to Key Performance Indicators (KPIs). Subject to change pending management approval, identified sample KPIs are:

1.	R&D portfolio of programs with KPIs	6.	Number of patents increased
2.	Delight the patient with quality outcomes and services	7.	Improved individual competency and capability
3.	Time-to-complete patient-centred solutions reduced	8.	Improved collaboration/workgroup performance
4.	Governance policy and procedures explicitly defined	9.	Improved internal cohesion with systems
5.	Knowledge flow to patient value accelerated	10.	Improved access to and quality of records (EHR)

Program 1 - Inventory and preserve knowledge: create taxonomy, identify records and define retention schedule.

- Goal 1: Enumerate and define all critical enterprise knowledge
- Goal 2: Reduce information loss across the enterprise.
- Goal 3: Ensure compliance with ISO 15489 for stored information.

Program 2 - Define viable operating environment: record patient. information, define patient projects, Manage facilities and resources.

- Goal 4: Enumerate and model all critical enterprise activities.
- Goal 5: Upgrade critical activities to improve outcomes.

Program 3 - Improve workforce competency and utilization.

- Goal 6: Update medical staff skills to leverage changing environments and technologies.

Program 4 - Leverage current and existing support systems: EHR, ERP, and CDS software, Telemedicine, HRM, Finance, and Legal.

- Goal 7: Minimize resource costs while insuring availability and capability of facilities and positive patient outcomes.

Program 5 – Optimize patient flow to wellness and facility utilization.

- Goal 8: Improve community health.
- Goal 9: Integrate in-hospital and out-of-hospital care within the region.

Threats by Program:

- Program 1: Gaps in information and incomplete, not validated records.
- Program 2: Lack of operating metrics to assure policy directives.
- Program 3: Inadequate skills to perform current and new tasks.
- Program 4: Lack of effective data collection to support patient. .diagnosis; poorly configured and deployed support system.
- Program 5: Inadequate operating data to affect optimal patient flow and critical staff, equipment, and facility usage.

Note: Project 5.6 "Simulate and Optimize Patient Flow to Wellness" under Program 5 occupies a significant number of pages. This book is an ongoing project; more work needs to be done to clarify and refine the Python simulations in Project 5.6 section. Also, this precedes work necessary to integrate it into Health IT and ERP systems. Both the Neural Network Simulation (NNS) and Discrete Event Simulation (DES) will require a great deal of data from those systems.

PROGRAM 1: KNOWLEDGE

Purpose: The goal is to create a streamlined, technology-enabled framework for healthcare operations, focusing on the organization and accessibility of critical knowledge, enhancing Electronic Health Records (EHRs), and leveraging system integrations to improve outcomes.

Key Concepts
- Document-Centric Knowledge Management:
    - Roles: Transform raw data into actionable insights, define processes, and organize information into retrievable taxonomies.
    - Categories: Knowledge, Transaction, Management, Capability, and External documents drive operational efficiency and compliance.
- Enterprise Taxonomy and Metadata:
    - Develop a taxonomy for critical documents as in Table 2-1.
    - Use Dublin Core metadata standards for categorization and retrieval.
    - Comply with ISO 15489 for document authenticity, reliability, integrity, and usability.
- Regulatory Compliance:
    - Ensure adherence to laws like HIPAA and Sarbanes-Oxley (SOX).
    - Develop records retention schedules and secure repositories.
- Healthcare System Integration:
    - Leverage Health IT systems (e.g., EPIC, Cerner) for data management.
    - Utilize AI for clinical decision support and discrete event simulations for resource optimization.
    - Define workflows for patient care, integrating diagnosis, treatment, and rehabilitation.
- Technical Framework:
    - Build secure IT and IoT infrastructure for data exchange and storage.
    - Enable collaboration with telecommunication systems.

Enterprise taxonomy (card catalog) classifies knowledge necessary to operate and govern the enterprise. For example, a marketing category may contain entities such as a news release template, a brochure template, a sales support guide and other categories such as Competitive Information and Voice of the Customer. Library scientists have a long history of collecting and classifying information / books. Computer software has evolved to develop taxonomy and ontology.

Competing on knowledge and leveraging intellectual assets is a critical component in the viability and profitability of an enterprise. A critical factor in supporting those objectives is for a firm to develop a taxonomy of its knowledge so that it can store, manage, locate, and (re)use it. Equally important in the taxonomy is monitoring and managing transaction documents that track progress of knowledge creation through explicitly defined process steps. For example, Sarbanes-Oxley Act (SOX) requires critical financial documents be available on-demand for the SEC, and also that their generation and validation be tracked and recorded.

Knowledge (KM)	Management	Transaction	Capability	External	Patient EHR
Market - Market Assessment - Client Literature - Stakeholder Mat'l - Client Profile - Client Fair Tasks	**Governance** - Policy/Guidelines - Finance/Acctg - Legal/Contracts - Security/Privacy - Audit Criteria	**Requests & POs** - Usage Forecast - Facility - Resource - Material - Specialist	**HRM Employee** - Experience - Education - Job classes - Skills	**Agreements** - Supplier - Benefactor - Customer - Leases - Real Estate	**Patient State** - Located - Transported - Accepted/Interviewed - Treated - Released
Develop - R&D Portfolio - Change Programs - R&D Projects - Business Cases - Prototypes	**Strategy** - Mission/vision - Goals/objectives - Budgets/Allocations - Pricing/Positioning - Completion Criteria	**Requirements** - Staff - Capability - Delivery - Resource - Material	**Technology** - Information - Communication - Automation - Computation	**Stakeholder** - Rules (ICD10) - Billing Req. - Requirements - Time-to-Pay - Dividends	**Patient Portfolio** - Diagnosis - Tests - ICD 10 condition - Interventions - Rehabilitations
Purchase - Supplier History - Resource Lists - RFOs/Quotes - Contracts - Inventories	**Change Req.** - Studies - Change Portfolio - New Capabilities - Projects/Milestones - Completion Criteria	**Schedule** - Facility - Patient - Bottlenecks - Idle Capacity - Back Schedule	**Financial** - Cash - Inventory - Market Valuation - Accounting - Billing	**Supplier** - P.O.s - Invoices - Strategy - D&B Supplier	**Patient EHR** **SOAP/OODA** • Financial/ICD10 Billing • Patient demographics • Progress notes • Vital signs
Deliver - Patient Portfolios - Facility Utilization - Quality Criteria - Delivery Criteria	**Operations** - Directives - Forecasts - Audit/status reports - Incentives	**Work Approvals** - Tollgate Sign-off - Test Acceptance - Patient registration - Portfolio verify	**Property/Equip.** - Real Estate - IT networks - Clinical Devices - Tools/Furniture	**Competitors** - Strategy - Ranking - Outcomes - D&B Rating	• Medical histories • Diagnoses • Medications • Immunization dates • Allergies • Radiology images
Maintain - Support Guidelines - Client Support Cost - Client Profile - Renewal Plans - Assessment Report	**Measures** - Velocity - Outcomes - Quality - Cost	**Status** - Portfolio Progress - Process History - Maint. History	**Supplier Profile** - Status - Capability - Capacity - Product/Service	**Government** - Laws - Standards - Regulations	• Lab and test results • Audio, video, plots • Record Inventories • Facility Utilization • Patient monitor data (hospital & home)
	Models - Tollgate Review - Collaboration - Portfolio - Beer's VSM	**History** - Inventory Levels - Available Resource - Failure Notification - Transaction Reports - Outcome Data	**KM & IP** - Methods - Deliverables - Patents / IP - 12 Pts Assess	**Economy** - Market indicators - Global Politics - WEF GCI **Environmental Health & Safety**	**Patient Operations** - Patient Scheduling - Staff Schedules - Staff Assignments - Treatment Workflows - Program Reports

Table 2-1 Enterprise/Hospital Document Hierarchy

Document Categories

Once a high-level taxonomy is established, the next step is to derive a minimal set of categories for the information that is accessed to generate the visible critical documents. This comes from millions of documents that currently reside in the enterprise paper and electronic file system. Table 2-1 illustrates a sample taxonomy of categories; most of the categories will apply to hospitals as well as many major companies (except EHR). Once a taxonomy is defined, metadata is added to further classify information. To manually build a high-level enterprise taxonomy:

- Identify Critical Documents and their lifecycles.
- Develop the taxonomy structure by understanding critical documents necessary to create value and operate the enterprise.
- Allow for ad-hoc documents in each category.
- Expand the taxonomy with critical documents required for governance, compliance and operation.
- Expand the taxonomy with knowledge based on core competencies and imbedded in processes and systems.
- Categorize content and place the pointers to the documents in the hierarchical structure – e.g. build a file folder structure in a file system and put critical documents in folders or install and configure a document management system.
- Determine how to present information that helps find it.
- Use taxonomy software to sub-categorize unstructured data.
- Process concepts to develop clusters of related concepts or documents.
- Develop taxonomy substructure.
- Decide if major classifications need to be restructured.
- Add sub-categories to the revised enterprise taxonomy.
- Add to the Dublin Core metadata that identifies a document's creator, subject, description, publisher, contributor, date, type, format, identifier, source, language, relation, coverage, and rights.

Governance, Records, Regulation and Retention

Sarbanes-Oxley Act (SOX) holds corporate officers and Sr. managers criminally liable for failing to:

- Conduct business according to strict interpretations of the Generally Accepted Accounting Principles..
- Make accurate and timely reports as prescribed by SEC.
- Properly manage and maintain corporate records..

Regulatory Compliance

ARMA (Association of Records Managers & Administrators) defines a record as recorded information that supports the activity of the business or organization that created it. If a document is a record, it must be identified as such and have a defined retention/destruction period.

Compliance maintains records to provide evidence of a firm's governance obligations. SOX regulatory documents are categorized under External/ Government Documents. SOX is focused on executives, governance and accounting; it requires companies to provide auditable proof that corporate records for reported financials are managed and maintained accurately.

Complying with the SEC Act of 1934 assures the necessary controls and procedures to gather, analyze, and disclose all information required by the SEC. However, SOX gives the SEC new authority to prosecute corporate officers and managers for inept corporate record management that can result in fines, and/or imprisonment.

Case law defines corporate records to include email, files on disk, voice mail, hand-written notes, paper or electronic drafts and renditions of documents. A company must demonstrate continual administration and execution of its corporate record retention policy to verify that its reporting results in thorough and consistent management of all documentation.

SOX compliance could bring corporate benefits:
- Faster, simpler access to critical business information,
- Lower document distribution costs,
- Accelerated workflow: measurable business environment,
- Protection of company intellectual property.

ISO 15489 (ISO: International Standards Organization) defines a document as recorded information or an object, which can be treated as a unit. A document is a piece of information in any media (paper, cassette, video, photograph, microfilm, etc.) Ad-hoc documents are temporary and are used for personal or workgroup productivity. Critical documents have lasting value, are defined by business process, and require different lifecycles. Records are critical documents that must be retained for specific legal, regulatory, or business requirements.

A record should correctly reflect what was communicated or decided or what action was taken. An ISO15489 compliant record must have:

- Authenticity: proved to be what it claims to be and created by the person at the time claimed.
- Reliability: trusted as a full and accurate content.
- Integrity: complete and unaltered.
- Usability: can be located, retrieved, presented, and interpreted.

Medical Documents and Records (see Appendix A)

Documents (and records) play a critical role in patient flow to positive outcomes. The interrelated, concurrent support cycles of Knowledge, Document, Workflow and Management support every business and medical process.

The Electronic Health Record (EHR) is the electronic file that contains the systematic documentation of a single patient's medical history of care across time. The medical record includes "notes" entered over time by health care professionals, recording observations and administration of drugs and therapies, orders for the administration of drugs and therapies, test results, x-rays, reports, etc. The maintenance of complete and accurate medical records is enforced by certification for healthcare providers.

The medical record serves as the central repository for planning patient care and documenting communication among patient and health care provider and professionals contributing to the patient's care. A medical record for inpatient care can include admission notes, on-service notes, progress notes (SOAP notes), preoperative notes, operative notes, postoperative notes, procedure notes, delivery notes, postpartum notes, and discharge notes.

SOAP note (Subjective, Objective, Assessment, Plan) is the method that health care providers use to write notes in a patient's chart. SOAP notes are placed in EHRs by phall medical personnel.

Subjective component: Initially it is a direct quote by the patient as to the purpose of the visit. Initially, a physician will take a History of Present Illness (HPI) to describe the patient's current condition. It will include all pertinent symptoms under review of body systems, pertinent medical/surgical history, family history, social history, medications, drug, alcohol, caffeine use, smoking status, physical activity level and allergies.

Objective component: documents what the healthcare provider observes or measures from the patient's current presentation including:

- Vital signs and measurements, such as weight.
- Results from past laboratory/diagnostic tests.
- Findings from physical examinations.

Assessment Component is a diagnosis from the medical visit and a summary note of a patient's main symptoms/ diagnosis including a list of other possible diagnoses in order of most to least likely. The assessment includes possible causes of patient problems, progress since the last visit and progress toward patient goals from the physician's perspective. A pharmacist's SOAP note assessment identifies what drug related/ induced problem is likely and the reason behind it. This includes risk factors, assessments of the need for therapy, current therapy, and therapy options.

Plan Component identifies the intervention to treat the patient's concerns - such as ordering further labs, radiological work up, referrals, procedures to perform, medications, surgery, education, goals of therapy and patient-specific drug and disease-state monitoring parameters. For patients with multiple health problems that are addressed in the SOAP note, a plan is developed for each problem and is numbered accordingly based on severity and urgency for therapy; often Assessment and Plans are grouped together.

Program 1 Knowledge Projects

Problem: A significant amount of critical information is lost over time, while EHRs are often populated with incomplete and inaccurate data.
Purpose: Define current state, validation, and availability challenges of EHRs and critical operational data to inventory and preserve knowledge.
Objective: Program focuses on inventorying, structuring, and preserving critical knowledge to support enterprise operations and compliance.
Goal 1: Enumerate and define critical enterprise knowledge:
- **Target 1.1**: Ensure all knowledge is uniformly defined without conflicting information.
- **Target 1.2**: Align critically important areas with national guidelines.

Goal 2: Reduce information loss across the enterprise:
- **Target 1.3**: Increase information sharing and collaboration.

Goal 3: Ensure compliance with ISO 15489 for stored information:
- **Target 1.4**: Validate clinical and long-term care data to ensure conciseness and completeness.

Context

Loss of information leads to duplication of knowledge work and renders clinical decision support systems ineffective which is addressed by:

- Continuously evaluating information structures.
- Creating a comprehensive taxonomy.
- Defining a validation process to capture critical knowledge.
- Focusing solely on entities within the firm (excluding external areas).

Ongoing Actions

- Inventory information gaps within a knowledge process model.
- Classify enterprise information within a knowledge taxonomy.
- Validate all information in EHRs to ensure ISO 15489 compliance.
- Revise the SOAP framework to enhance analysis with AI algorithms.

Key Performance Indicators Metrics	Weight
Number of mutually exclusive knowledge categories identified	30%
Number of gaps in required information, records, knowledge	30%
Percentage of records validated as complete and accurate	20%
Percentage of conflicting descriptions resolved	20%

Threats and Risks

- Lack of information to assist with appropriate planning.
- Excessive time spent "finding" critical knowledge, causing delays.
- Insufficient time spent "discovering" critical knowledge areas, leading to incomplete taxonomy.

Team: Library Scientist; Computer Scientist; Process Engineer

PROJECT CHARTERS

Project 1.1: Language Conflict Resolution

Problem: Critical knowledge is miscommunicated due to inconsistent naming conventions for the same entities.

Purpose: Ensure enterprise knowledge is accurate and complete.

Objective: Standardize critical information naming conventions across the medical region.

Future State: Nurse Paul, previously hindered by inconsistent terminology is now finding wound care information quickly that is accurate and relevant due to standardized language across the region.

Actions and Deliverables

- **Culture**: Negotiate consistent naming conventions.
- **Content**: Identify identical document types with but different names.
- **Process**: Publish a discrepancy list and resolved naming conventions.
- **Risk:** Information security not HIPPA compliant.

Metrics

- Time to access critical records and information.
- Number of patients accessing appropriate information.
- Monthly information request volume.

Benefits
- Concise communication among medical personnel.
- Reduced confusion regarding information accuracy.

Project 1.2: Define Knowledge Taxonomy

Problem: Critical knowledge is unavailable, incomplete, or inaccurate.

Purpose: Improve access to critical documents and records for clinical operations and patient care.

Objective: Develop a comprehensive taxonomy for better information access across the region.

Future State: Paramedic Ann responds to an elder's emergency signal. With access to accurate EHRs, she identifies a previous TIA and coordinates timely and effective intervention with a virtual ER physician.

Actions and Deliverables
- **Culture**: Train personnel to access newly categorized information.
- **Content**: Develop a list of mutually exclusive knowledge categories.
- **Process**: Define a comprehensive taxonomy.
- **Architecture**: Establish a system-wide taxonomy.
- **Infrastructure**: Ensure information is accessible across the region.
- **Risk:** Information not HIPPA compliant.

Metrics
- Time to access critical records and information.
- Number of patients accessing appropriate information.
- Monthly information request volume.

Benefits
- Patients access progress reports on diagnosis, intervention, and rehab.
- Reduced information duplication.
- Less verbal communication for previously documented issues.

Project 1.3: Define Records Retention Schedule

Problem: Records are not explicitly defined, leading to confusion about their classification and retention periods.

Purpose: Ensure all records are identified and retained for appropriate durations as required by law.

Objective: Comply with federal and state laws for archiving, preserving, and securing records.

Future State: Records Manager Winston's team ensures proper archiving and email management. This reduces legal risks, such as discovery of inappropriate comments during litigation.

Actions and Deliverables
- **Culture**: Train staff on records management rules and email usage.
- **Content**: Define a comprehensive records retention schedule.
- **Process**: Identify documents that qualify as legal records.
- **Architecture**: Provide secure online access for authorized records.
- **Infrastructure**: Maintain a secure repository for records, preventing unauthorized modifications.
- **Risk**: Records insecurity and improper email management.

Metrics
- Number of ISO 15489-compliant records.
- Compliance with HIPAA for record storage.
- Retention schedules for all critical records.

Benefits
- Reduced litigation risks from improper record handling.
- Increased awareness of information obligations among staff.

Project 1.4: Establish Tollgate Review Process
Problem: Inaccurate EHR and ERP data hinder diagnosis and staff scheduling.
Purpose: Establish policies and procedures for auditing documents.
Objective: Ensure all information complies with ISO 15489 standards.
Future State: CMO Clara Barton ensures staff access to accurate, timely information to improve scheduling, minimize costs, and optimize resource utilization.

Actions and Deliverables
- **Culture**: Train staff in tollgate review methods.
- **Content**: Subject all information and records to review.
- **Process**: Develop and publish a tollgate review process.
- **Architecture**: Use collaboration software for virtual reviews.
- **Infrastructure**: Leverage telecommunication for dispersed teams.
- **Risk**: Records inaccuracy.
- Number of ISO 9000-compliant records.
- Compliance with HIPAA for record storage.
- Retention schedules for all critical records.

Benefits
- EHRs are ISO15489 compliant supporting more accurate diagnosis from CDS and AI.
- Resources are reassigned based on projects progress and requirements.

PROGRAM 2: PROCESS

An Introduction to Processes

Processes are the practical application of enterprise knowledge, reflected in repeatable tasks to achieve key functions. They transform knowledge into action and are unique to each organization. However, a generic process model can be defined for industries such as healthcare and manufacturing. These models enable organizations to:

- Specify critical document linkages within and between processes.
- Define processes as projects using project management methods.
- Monitor document flow and analyze variance through process histories.
- Identify bottlenecks and inefficiencies in document formats and flows.

Adopting a document-centric perspective facilitates process modeling and simulation, offering clarity in how processes interact.

The Core Process Model for Healthcare

Processes defined by documents create the framework to:

Market	to educated customers with timely, accurate proposals.
Develop	desirable, easy-to-build products defined by Design Drawings.
Purchase	resources from trusted, reliable suppliers using Documents to facilitate transactions.
Deliver	quality, low cost products, capability, and services delivered on-time, based on transaction documents.
Maintain	customers in a way that ensures continued business using Maintenance Manuals, Scheduling and Account History documents.

In healthcare, medical staff use a variety of less structured documents so that in many cases the success or failure of patient outcomes is not well-understood, precisely because of inadequate structure and non-ISO15489 electronic health records. Evolving to comprehensive document structures and ISO15489 compliant health records and explicitly defined ISO 9001 compliant process workflows present an opportunity to improve patient outcomes and lower cost.

To illustrate how knowledge is delivered to a hospital's value chain, the next level of the generic model is Figure 3-1 for healthcare. Taking a project view of process with documents as their milestones creates an explicit definition of "the way work is structured." The document model of core processes has great value in revealing the linkages that enable processes to operate concurrently rather than serially. All core processes must work together to create a successful enterprise. At a high level, Figure 3-1 depicts the processes in providing healthcare to the community.

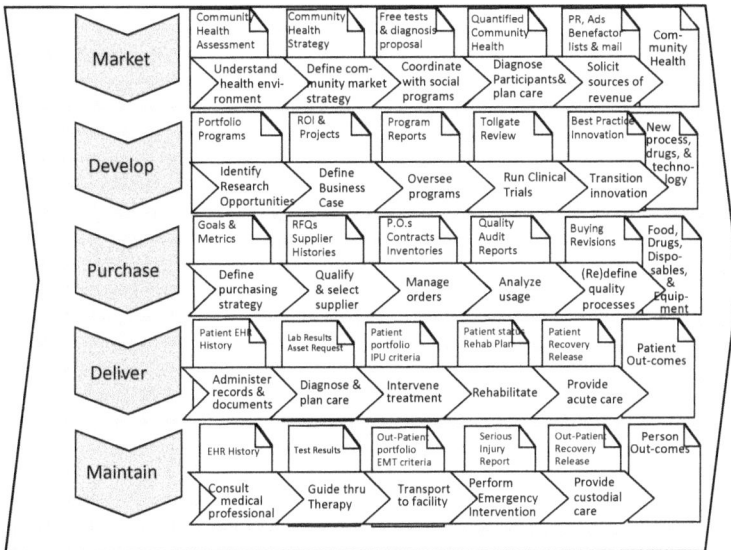

Figure 3-1: *Each health system process interacts with the others.*

Marketing Processes and Document Linkages

The top row of arrows in Figure 3-1 represents the marketing core process model. Because a healthy community and cost containment are important to healthcare providers, marketing has the task of deciding what potential patients need, not just when they get sick, but how to keep them as healthy as possible so that if they do get sick, they have a better chance to recover. Marketing must involve the entire organization in developing service requirements for the community not just in delivery services to "fix" ailments. It must partner with physicians to identify services for quality hospital care and emergency service as well as home healthcare providers to ensure surrounding community members are better served in a reasonable time frame and at a competitive cost.

Marketing should understand what patients will need in the future and educate them about maintaining healthy habits and the benefits of hospital services. Market documents must define what the development team must produce and how much time they have to bring it to market.

Development Processes and Document Linkages
The second row in Figure 3-1 indicates the development process and its documents. Because the document view is the only constant during the R&D stage, it is the only way to develop a process model for this activity.

Development assembles a program that transitions the hospital from its current to a future state. This may involve improved billing processes to reduce the number of billing rejections from insurers and Medicare, improved flow of patients through the ER, improved utilization of critical facilities such as operating theaters, optimize the allocation of beds, minimize inventories, assure delivery of disposables, maximize the flow of lab results, and many other processes in the delivery of medical services.

Records and Resource Management software can help to improve the quality of care but only if it is delivered along with changed processes and staff education, which must be part of the development plan.

Development must also create a portfolio of projects for the development and installation of new medical equipment and technology. Further, it must have research portfolios of all new drugs and techniques and tests being sponsored by the healthcare facility.

Purchasing Processes and Document Linkages
Figure 3-1 shows purchasing between develop and deliver. To reduce cost-for-delivery, purchasing must take an active role in both processes rather than be just a service organization. In a patient to wellness outcome environment, it is critical that the document network allows purchasing to facilitate delivery of drugs, disposables and new capabilities.

Purchasing must develop a strategy that supports delivery of both medical and non-medical supplies from a qualified supplier. Qualification certifies suppliers by auditing their key processes and process management to ensure that their practices are compatible with the hospital demands. Purchasing involves supplier selection, price negotiation, claims negotiation, and terms and conditions as part of the hospital supply process.

Delivery Processes and Document Linkages
The fourth row in Figure 3-1 illustrates the Deliver process and is derived from Michael Porter's theory of an Integrated Practice Unit (IPU). To coordinate development by different people in different areas at different times, it is essential that there is a common, comprehensive view of the hospital in place.

Figure 3-2 shows Porter's IPU processes modified using 6σ monitoring and change functions (in chapter 6) that supports both Deliver and Maintain.

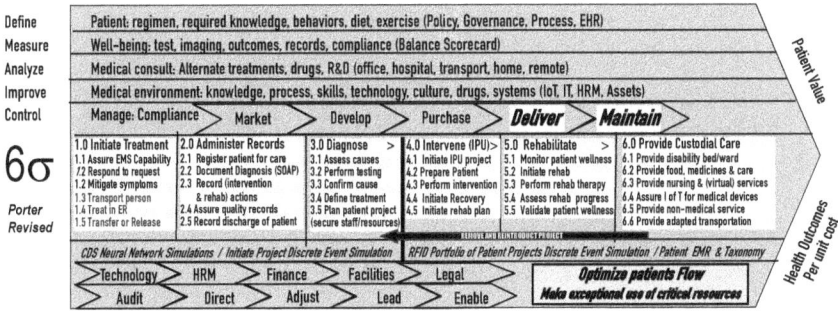

Figure 3-2: *Porter's Integrated Practice Unit Modified*

This common view allows document templates, macros and data structures to be effectively shared for both analysis and operation of medical systems. This use of 6σ in the healthcare context particularly allows bottom-up measurements of quality patient outcomes against cost of delivery. These measurements are further reflected in the top-down views shown as a Balanced Scorecard (in Chapter 4).

The list of attributes relates specifically to implementing business capabilities for 16 complex care areas shown are:

- Cancer
- Geriatrics
- Gynecology
- Nephrology
- Ophthalmology

- Cardiology & Heart Surgery
- Diabetes & Endocrinology
- Ear, Nose & Throat
- Gastroenterology & GI Surgery
- Neurology & Neurosurgery

- Orthopedics
- Pulmonology
- Psychiatry
- Rehabilitation
- Rheumatology
- Urology

Management of organizational complexity is dependent on effective, quality operations for these complex care areas which exist at the grassroots level of a healthcare organization. Modeling this complexity depends on using a process improvement framework, such as Lean 6σ, to manage and monitor the IPUs associated with each complex care area.

The 16 complex care areas are also the subject of the collaboration health check described earlier. Taken together, 6σ and the Porter IPU in Figure 3-3 are the basis for the processes associated with "Deliver" in Figure 3-2. In the implementation of Porter's IPU framework it may well end up with less than 16 complex care areas. However, in terms of optimizing organizational complexity, the elements of complex care areas are considered to be local as they reside at lower levels of the healthcare process model, which is of particular relevance to this book.

Maintenance Processes and Document Linkages
The details in the fifth row in figure 3-1 represent care in the home as well as care in emergencies. Maintain must treat out-patients in the community with what appears to be very similar to in-patient treatment in "Deliver." However, "Intervention" is much different and less intense than Porter's IPU hospital interventions. Chemotherapy, dialysis and simple surgery, may be done in out-patient settings.

Process improvement has been a fundamental underlying part of Federal mandates. Medicare ACOs (Accountable Care Organization) were created to improve the efficiency of the networks of hospitals and doctors that deliver services to Medicare patients and thereby lower the government's costs. In addition to a continuous process improvement program to reduce cost of care, the hospital pro-actively reaches out to their community patient enrollees to keep them healthy to avoid costly interventions later.

"ACOs are groups of doctors, hospitals, and other health care providers, who come together voluntarily to give coordinated high-quality care to their Medicare patients. The goal of coordinated care is to ensure that patients get the right care at the right time, while avoiding unnecessary duplication of services and preventing medical errors."

For "Maintain" in the model to work effectively, requires that the disparate out-patient services must share the same IT system and are much more dependent on telemedicine. Also, effectively coordinating a care team will require telemedicine to provide diagnosis, custodial care and out-patient progress tracking (Chapter 5).

VA Health System has 70,000 telemedicine visits/year and they declare how much it saves money in the largest health system in the United States. Medicare for the elderly and Medicaid for the poor pays for telemedicine services. Video conferences have been shown to be comparable to face-to-face in terms of diagnostic accuracy, patient acceptance, and cost.

Using telemedicine, an attending PA or paramedic in collaboration with a hospital ER physician can effectively diagnosis patient symptoms and provide the correct medical intervention and if necessary, arrange for EMS to transfer the patient to the most appropriate, nearest medical facility.

Custodial care for the elderly may benefit the most from coordinated out-patient team care and telemedicine. Consider that a mentally capable, frail elder in the home cannot perform many simple tasks (e.g. bathing, food preparation, shopping, etc.) necessary to maintain his or her independence.

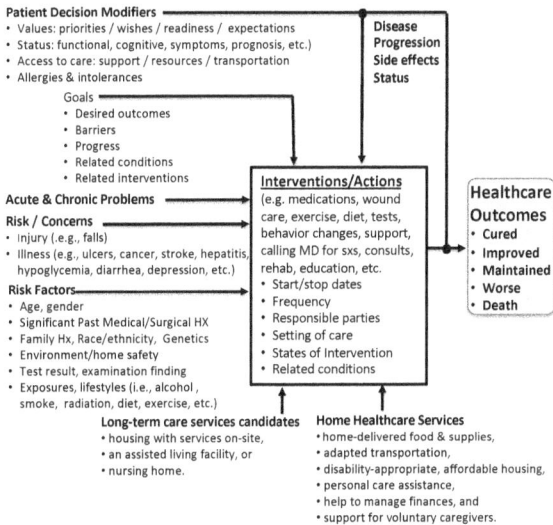

Patient Decision Modifiers
- Values: priorities / wishes / readiness / expectations
- Status: functional, cognitive, symptoms, prognosis, etc.)
- Access to care: support / resources / transportation
- Allergies & intolerances

Disease Progression Side effects Status

Goals
- Desired outcomes
- Barriers
- Progress
- Related conditions
- Related interventions

Acute & Chronic Problems

Risk / Concerns
- Injury (.e.g., falls)
- Illness (e.g., ulcers, cancer, stroke, hepatitis, hypoglycemia, diarrhea, depression, etc.)

Risk Factors
- Age, gender
- Significant Past Medical/Surgical HX
- Family Hx, Race/ethnicity, Genetics
- Environment/home safety
- Test result, examination finding
- Exposures, lifestyles (i.e., alcohol, smoke, radiation, diet, exercise, etc.)

Interventions/Actions (e.g. medications, wound care, exercise, diet, tests, behavior changes, support, calling MD for sxs, consults, rehab, education, etc.
- Start/stop dates
- Frequency
- Responsible parties
- Setting of care
- States of Intervention
- Related conditions

Healthcare Outcomes
- Cured
- Improved
- Maintained
- Worse
- Death

Long-term care services candidates
- housing with services on-site,
- an assisted living facility, or
- nursing home.

Home Healthcare Services
- home-delivered food & supplies,
- adapted transportation,
- disability-appropriate, affordable housing,
- personal care assistance,
- help to manage finances, and
- support for voluntary caregivers.

Figure 3-3: Elements of Elder and Custodial Care

Figure 3-3 reflects the elements of an elder care program under Maintain. In the past, this would require placing the elder in a nursing home, but now with telemedicine using Medicare PACE guidelines (Program of All-Inclusive Care for the Elderly), an attending spouse (also possibly frail) with daily visits from qualified care givers and visits from a paramedic in communication with a virtual physician, the elder can be cared for in his or her home, thereby improving quality of life at much lower cost of care. Emergency events both in an elder's home or in a senior care can be frequently handled by a paramedic and virtual physician eliminating the need for an expensive, traumatic transport and ER visit.

Services to support in home care:	Community Services for home care:
• Care coordination/case management navigation • Personal care (baths, nail cut, haircut, bed change) • Homemaker services (cleaning, cooking) • Home-delivered meals or food • Home reconfiguration (ramps, lighting, bathrooms) • Home hospice • Telephone reassurance and monitoring services • Connectivity Technologies • Emergency/urgent advice /non-medical issue help	• Meals at congregate sites • Adapted transportation • Help with legal and finances • Counselling to improve family dynamics • Friendly visitors and telephones • Socialization (call networks, neighbor visits, etc.) • Investigate abuse, fraud, neglect • Day adult care hospital services • Caregiver skills education, group support, respite • Medication management • Nursing: wound care, drugs, devices • Equipment rental and exchange

Telemedicine and OODA Loops: Fundamental to Diagnosis

Shewhart's (not Deming) PDSA cycle was the seminal work associated with most of analysis and change done in hospitals. However, its philosophy is built to analyze and change manufacturing processes that are explicitly defined with relatively stable cycle times and variation. Hospitals processes are not. Col. John Boyd's OODA (Observe, Orient, Decide, Act) loops is a better paradigm for documenting doctor/patient relationships. Boyd originally conceived OODA as a theory of warfare for jet fighters; it has subsequently been used to develop business strategy. It has been adopted by some in the medical community. OODA loop framework for decision-making in healthcare, complements traditional evidence-based approaches. This iterative process:

- Emphasizes intuitive, context-sensitive decision-making.
- Adapts to the complexities of human physiology and psychology.
- Links observations and actions to improve patient outcomes.

In Figure 3-4, Orientation shapes observation, shapes decision, shapes action and in turn, is shaped by the feedback and other phenomena coming into our sensing or observation window. Also note how the entire "loop" (not just orientation) is an ongoing many-sided implicit cross-referencing process of projection, empathy, correlation, and rejection.

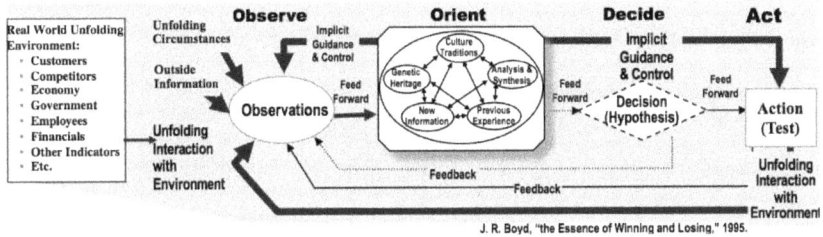

J. R. Boyd, "the Essence of Winning and Losing," 1995.

Figure 3-4: OODA Loop

Without generic heritage, cultural traditions, and previous experiences, one does not possess an implicit repertoire of psychophysical skills shaped by environments and changes that have been previously experienced. Without analysis and synthesis, across a variety of domains or across a variety of competing/independent channels of information, one cannot evolve new repertories to deal with unfamiliar phenomenon or unforeseen change.

Without many sided implicit cross-referencing processes of projection, empathy, correlation, and rejection, (across many different domains or channels of information), one cannot even do analysis and synthesis. Without OODA loops, one can neither sense, hence observe, thereby collect a variety of information for the above processes, nor decide as well as implement in accord with those processes.

EHRs and SOAP notes link many medical processes. Consequently, any global change to the medical process must be built around linkages/documents that define relationships between activities.

According to a new study published in JAMA Network Open which included 26 attendings and 24 residents, were given six case histories selected from a larger set of 105 real cases... Doctors who used and ignored ChatGPT had a median score of 76%. In comparison, the doctors who only used traditional resources had a median score of 74%... ChatGPT on its own outperformed both groups of doctors, with a median score of 90% for making a diagnosis and providing a reason.

Consider that AI in a Neural Network Simulation (NNS) acts like a super-fast OODA loop. In chapter 6, ChatGPT defined a Python program that used an NNS to determine the cause and intervention from patient symptoms. ChatGPT was then used to define a Python program that used Discrete Event Simulation to optimize a portfolio of patient flow to wellness through critical areas of the hospital.

Explicitly Defined, Validated Process
The value of "enterprise knowledge" is frequently documents, which must be validated. Critical to an explicitly defined, validated process are Work Instructions and Rules. In poorly defined processes, work instructions do not exist and frequently rules are ignored in order to finish quickly. In this case finishing quickly may mean sending wrong information downstream so that all of the work has to be redone once the errors are discovered. Process validation is critical to accelerating the "total" process.

Understanding process is key to establishing economic value added or return on equity as a result of changing a knowledge environment. This is accomplished by monitoring and measuring the rate at which knowledge and innovation flow to customer defined value (patient flow to wellness).

A project vision of leadership is tied directly to what business processes must accomplish. With the project vision come initiatives to achieve it. In addition, process-oriented leadership includes the allocation of necessary resources to adequately support business process. **Project management** must be PMI (Project Management Institute) compliant and utilize work breakdown structures to clearly define accurate timelines, activities, tasks, dependencies, and project team resources to deliver a result.

Program 2 Process Projects
Problem: Management has a limited understanding of how knowledge flows through operating processes to create positive outcomes.
Purpose Improve operational efficiency by optimizing knowledge flow within healthcare processes to enhance patient outcomes.

Objective: Create a comprehensive model for continuous evaluation and performance improvement.

Goal 4. Enumerate and model all critical enterprise activities:
- **Target 2.1**: Define all critical health system activities in a high-level iDEF0 function model.
- **Target 2.2**: Identify activities with large gaps in information and skills.

Goal 5. Upgrade critical activities to improve outcomes:
- **Target 2.3**: Monitor, audit, and summarize all activities on a management evaluation dashboard.

Ongoing Program Actions
- Identify key areas within the organization and interview relevant personnel.
- Address information and skill gaps in activities through a functional knowledge process model.
- Synthesize disparate models into a unified organizational model guided by The Document Methodology.
- Propose two interim and one a future state to transform a health system.

Key Performance Indicators Metric	Weight
Percentage of the organization embraced by the model	30%
Problems preventing effective knowledge flow to value	10%
Percentage of resolved problems affecting knowledge flow	30%
Time to implement an "almost as-is" model	30%

Threats and Risks
- Lack of inventories and information to support planning.
- Excessive time spent "discovering" critical knowledge areas, causing delays and cost overruns.
- Insufficient effort to discover critical knowledge areas, leading to incomplete taxonomy.

PROJECT CHARTERS
Project 2.1: Define Knowledge/Process Model
Problem: No comprehensive overview exists of how the health system operates to treat patients and provide long-term care.
Purpose: Define how knowledge flows through process to patient wellness.
Objectives: Document knowledge flow for treatment and long-term care.
Future State: The Chief Medical Officer (CMO) has access to a dashboard offering statistics on medical provision flow, facility scheduling (e.g., ORs, beds, lab work), and personnel allocation.
Actions and Deliverables
- **Culture**: Gain consensus from interviewed personnel that the model represents operations.

- **Content**: Create a high-level view of knowledge flow leading to positive patient outcomes.
- **Process**: Identify key organizational areas and interview personnel. Synthesize interviews into a validated enterprise model.
- **Architecture**: Define system support for current knowledge flow and identify improvement opportunities.
- **Infrastructure**: Telecommunications, IT servers, mobile devices.
- **Risk:** Interviewees may not fully represent organizational breadth.

Metrics
- Time to complete validated knowledge/process model.
- Number of interviewees agreeing the model is comprehensive.
- Depth of process hierarchy (three or more levels).

Benefits: Improved understanding of how all organizational components interact to treat patients and provide long-term care.

Project 2.2: Identify Pathologies and Gaps

Problem: Staff struggles to access information necessary for their roles.
Purpose: Resolve bottlenecks and gaps in information flow using the document process model.
Objectives: Streamline knowledge flow to achieve positive patient outcome.
Future State: Nurses can access SOAP notes for patients with similar conditions, enabling quicker resolution of questions about patient monitoring data.

Actions and Deliverables
- **Culture**: Educate staff and build consensus on solution benefits.
- **Content**: Develop proposed future states in three steps.
- **Process**: Perform gap/risk analysis, identify bottlenecks, evaluate alternative resolutions, and propose a roadmap.
- **Architecture**: Use modeling, risk analysis and AI software.

Risks: Lack of consensus among consulted personnel.

Metrics
- Time to complete future state knowledge/process model.
- Level of consensus on the proposed roadmap.

Benefits: Staff agreement and advocacy for the transformation.

Project 2.3: Propose and Negotiate Future State

Problem: Staff acknowledge the benefits of a proposed future state but require assurance about its feasibility.
Purpose: Define a portfolio of programs detailing costs, timelines, and resources for achieving the future state.
Objectives: Define policies, goals, objectives, and a portfolio to transform healthcare and senior care in the region.
Future State: Management can monitor and adjust operations based on knowledge flow, improving policy-setting and organizational transformation.

Actions and Deliverables

- **Culture**: Communicate models and gain consensus on project responsibilities.
- **Content**: Propose policies and procedures to guide the organization towards milestones.
- **Process**: Define criteria to measure performance and propose an ideal future state model.
- **Architecture**: Project management and portfolio dashboard software.
- **Infrastructure**: Dashboard displays, telecom, and ISP servers.

Risk: Difficulty achieving consensus on criteria and responsibilities.
Metrics: Time and cost to complete the proposal.
Benefits: Staff agreement and advocacy for the transformation.

Project 2.4: Manage Process Environment

Problem: No overview exists of how the health system operates to treat patients and provide long-term care.
Purpose: Optimize operations by leveraging knowledge flow through them.
Objectives: Use knowledge flow statistics for patient care and long-term care to optimize operations.
Future State: The CMO has access to a dashboard providing statistics on medical provision flow, facility scheduling, and personnel allocation.

Actions and Deliverables

- **Culture**: Train management to interpret and act on dashboard statistics.
- **Content**: Create a dashboard of statistics for senior medical staff to evaluate system-wide operations.
- **Process**: Model a network describing all aspects of medical support.
- **Architecture**: Use collaboration and portfolio software for virtual reviews across regions.
- **Infrastructure**: Telecommunications and IT server access.
- **Risk:** Inaccurate statistics may lead to poor decisions.

Metrics

- Cost of operation.
- Compliance with HIPAA for record storage.
- Retention schedules for critical records.

Benefits

- Reduced litigation risks from improper record handling.
- Enhanced staff awareness of their information management obligations.

PROGRAM 3: MANAGE ENTERPRISE

Documents Provide Facts to Manage People

Objective: To optimize healthcare systems through robust management processes, leveraging document-driven strategies, performance metrics, and technology integration. The focus is on empowering employees, enabling innovation, and improving operational efficiency.

TDM's management model bridges the process models (Chapter 3), the systems model (Chapter 5), and the change model (Chapter 6), dynamically linking the initiation and completion of key knowledge and transaction documents. These documents, embodying the state of enterprise processes, become invaluable inputs for performance analysis.

People, who are educated to manage and change processes with facts from systems that summarize transaction documents, are able to:

Lead by effectively allocating resources based on facts.

Improve by changing processes, products and services in response to markets.

Direct by profitably producing products and services with processes that are fine-tuned to resolve bottlenecks by evaluating status and performance documents.

Audit by assessing variation of processes, products and services through real time monitoring of the velocity and content of all value-added documents.

Enable by supporting core processes with document systems that automate and accelerate document flow.

Figure 4-1 shows the documents in the relationship between the management and enterprise models. The word "system" is used because each of the four management components contained in Management System 1 are also found within Management Systems 2 through 5, the higher-level systems that affect it. Each level in the organization is managed with the same component systems, making this a recursive system definition of management process. Stafford Beer identified these component systems as a Viable System Model (VSM) in his book: "Brain of the Firm."

Circles of Causality Relate Documents

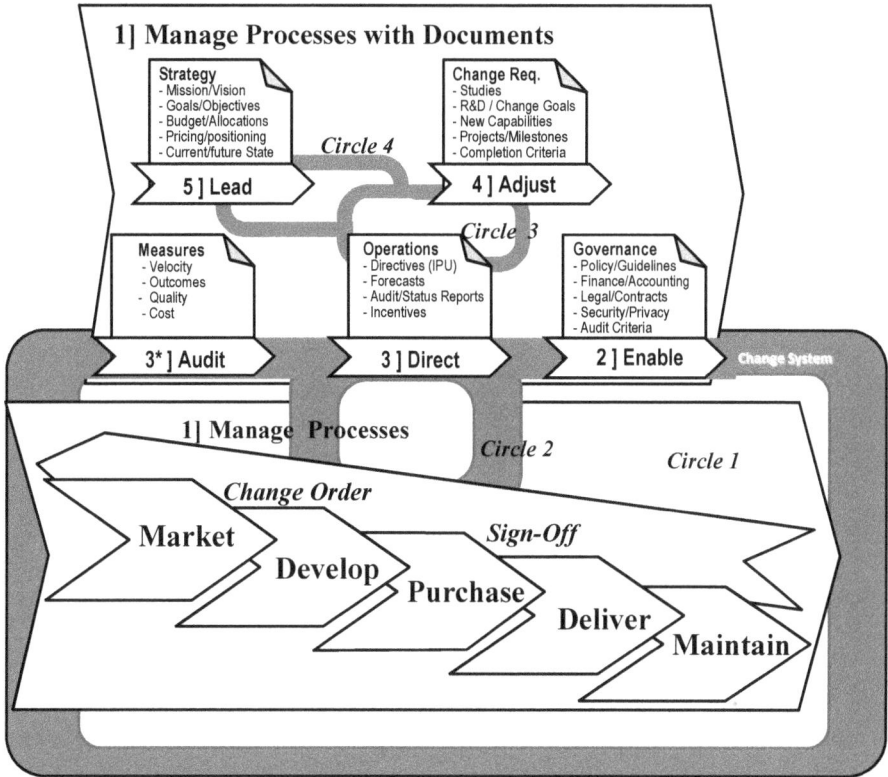

Figure 4-1: *Four circles of causality (+1: external environment)*

Management System 1: Manage Core Processes (on circles 1 & 2)

Management System 1 focuses on *implementation* of the core processes of a business, each of which is comprised of physically and technologically distinct tasks. These processes are an organization's building blocks for creating valuable products and services for its customers. Management System 1 views the totality of managing these individual core processes and their sub-processes. For example, the process of directing order fulfillment must be done within the context of improving the customer satisfaction, response and cost parameters that will enable the leadership strategies of capturing market share.

Management System 2: Enable (on circle 1)

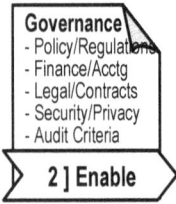

Governance
- Policy/Regulations
- Finance/Acctg
- Legal/Contracts
- Security/Privacy
- Audit Criteria

> 2] Enable >

Management System 2 *coordinates* core processes and sub-processes, how they relate to one another and with what constraints. To the extent that this system is supported by transaction documents and statistics resulting from a project view of process, people self-direct their activities.

To enable a process on circle 1 it must be:

Guided by procedures which assure *operations.*

Populated by people with competencies to perform *tasks.*

Systematized with a project view using the *support systems.*

Automated to accelerate performance with *technology.*

Facilitated by the physical *work environment.*

Governance Documents, which are *systematized* by the Support Systems, provide the information structure to empower people to act autonomously and collaboratively within an enterprise. Guidelines, HRM policy, budgets and transaction documents provide this structure.

For example, in executing the order fulfillment process, documents relating to credit status and guidelines must be readily available to support decision-making based on facts.

As organizational hierarchy is flattened, the related business processes must absorb complexity originally controlled by other levels of the organization. Unless that complexity can be simplified with a supportive management system, the result will be a chaotic work environment. Avoiding this requires job redesign and training so that the staff at all levels can improve and operate new core processes supported by transaction documents placing accountability closer to the action, where it belongs.

Management System 3: Direct on circles 1, 2, 3

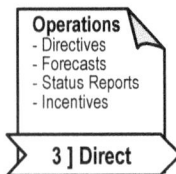

Operations
- Directives
- Forecasts
- Status Reports
- Incentives

> 3] Direct >

Management System 3 controls the *cohesion* of internal operations between core process management units to:

- Enforce regulations and systems (circle 1).
- Intervene to correct faults (circle 2).
- Deploy change to alleviate bottlenecks (circle 3).

The goals of Direct include insuring sufficient revenue to operate and improve the business, rewarding good performance, and correcting bad performance, whether that bad performance is due to the process itself or how it is being done. For example, misdiagnosis; can create a bottleneck in the use of critical equipment or facility that must be addressed.

Traditionally, this management system depended on a hierarchical command-and-control approach. This type of approach is less effective in today's fast-changing environment, but the management function itself is even more important. The current wealth of an enterprise is completely dependent on how it directs its operations.

As hospitals face an aging demographic and expand their virtual coverage to deal with rural patients, their focus changes from ensuring repeatable, day-to-day efficiency to ensuring effectiveness of rapid change.

The management system for improving processes becomes more prominent and increasingly influences the management systems for directing them. As businesses define organizational and product changes faster, Direct must not only direct current processes, but deploy new systems such as telemedicine to change the operating environment.

Knowledge documents provide the basic background for management systems to direct and improve processes, while transaction documents must contain the statistics to support efficient operations.

Management System 3*: Audit on circle 1

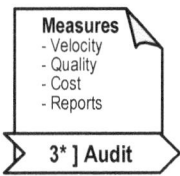

Measures
- Velocity
- Quality
- Cost
- Reports

▷ 3*] Audit ▷

Audit ensures that System 3 directives are carried out and System 2 governance is adhered to. The audit system inspects operating capability by evaluating costs, timing, and quality related to established metrics.

The Audit function of management is more complex as managers must manage many more people than in the past. It is simply not possible to confer continuously with all direct reports. Statistical Process Control (SPC) can be a partial solution. However, unless facts are available to summarize and analyze resource usage, process progress, and people's productivity, a manager must guess at key issues.

Process audit documents differ from financial audits. Most commonly, they are the statistical summary documents that result from continuously monitoring the progress of documents through individual tasks of processes. According to Deming, they provide necessary information to assess the variation and flaws in the process that allows continuous reduction of flaws, variation and process cycle time.

The facts required to manage reside in transaction documents. The key to meaningful management audit lies in monitoring the discrete deliverables of a process as projects defined by their transaction documents. Statistical summaries can identify process variation and bottlenecks in the current business process, which can accelerate completion of deliverables.

The reward system is also important and must be supported by broadly understood, clear, simple metrics in an enterprise culture that supports the search for better decision making and policy setting.

Management System 4: Adjust (on circle 3)
Management System 4 reinvents and plans the deployment of new processes based on intelligence derived from internal operating statistics and market evaluations.

Change Req.
- Studies
- R&D / Change Goals
- New Capabilities
- Projects/Milestones
- Completion Criteria

4] Adjust

For example, hospitals attempt to cut their time-to-wellness dramatically. Because healthcare environments are complex, a hospital's future wealth is heavily dependent on the effectiveness of the continuous improvement process.

Federal regulations, healthcare regulations, patents, new equipment capability, economic indicator reports, and wellness demographics are examples of events that influence requirements for change.

Critical documents associated with the Adjust process are those that represent the enterprise's translation of its future business vision into detailed specifications of deliverables. Given these specifications, additional documents define the projects, resources and schedules required to create the processes and facilities by which these products and services will be provided.

The Adjust component of management must occur at every level of the organization. The documents associated with the Improve component include project and problem definitions and the identification of solutions. There are several ways to assign a value to this activity financially, including increased market valuation, quicker process time cycles, improved profitability and reduced cost.

Management System 5: Lead (on circle 4 & 3)

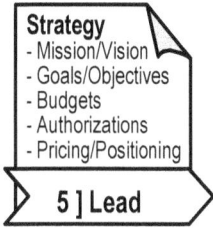

Strategy
- Mission/Vision
- Goals/Objectives
- Budgets
- Authorizations
- Pricing/Positioning

5] Lead

Management System 5 *leads* by monitoring and prioritizing conflict between improving and directing the enterprise to ensure smooth operation. The intervention on circle 3 provides the overall focus and direction for Systems 3 and 4. Leadership provides the overall focus and direction for those engaged in improving or directing the process to insure current and future profitability.

Resource allocation becomes the vehicle for structuring how change and operations are arbitrated. Leadership is facilitated by strong vision and mission statements, which can be communicated and understood not just by senior management but also by everyone in the organization. The vision must be a process mission statement, which employees can apply to their individual task.

As business and market demands accelerate, it is important to recognize that more resources must be given to those initiatives that are focused on building processes and structures that adapt effectively. A principal component of leadership is exercising the judgment to decide how much of the corporate resources to allocate to existing operations versus how much to allocate to proposed new products and processes.

Empowered Practitioners and Fact-Based Management
Management systems rely on empowered employees by:
- Encouraging innovation while maintaining output quality.
- Providing training and broaden the knowledge base.
- Leveraging document systems to disseminate critical information across the organization.

Fact-based management ensures informed decision-making by leveraging transaction data from clearly defined processes. Supported by workflow systems, management relies on:

- Milestone documents to track progress.
- Predictions for time-to-completion and resource allocation.
- Scheduling and monitoring to measure success.

In the past, the emphasis was on achieving a high degree of proficiency at a particular task or machine. Today, it's more important that staff expedite the completion of specific processes and emphasize responsiveness to customers and product and/or service quality.

Physician Competency with Telemedicine and AI

Chapter 2, 3 and 5 present the impact of telemedicine and information technology on out-patient and elderly care in a community of disparate caregivers. However, impact on clinical practice itself has proven far more challenging than the technology or patient acceptance where physicians have a high workload, and adding any more work is not possible.

The cost of introducing telemedicine equipment as well as artificial intelligence software into the office is formidable. In the ideal situation, without cost or staff concerns, the patient care can be much better when utilizing telemedicine and AI for diagnosis and treatment.

In the USA Veterans Health System, doctors on staff claim telemedicine actually takes less time. A well-coordinated telemedicine clinic is very efficient with almost no delay between patients. For an office physician with proper access to technology, the overhead costs of telemedicine visits are negligible when compared to cost of facilities and staff.

If telemedicine is left to the singular efforts of a physician, the task is very difficult. In the USA, there is a strong movement for telemedicine to be freestanding and not managed by the personal physician. This can certainly be seen as a threat to the sanctity of physician-patient relations. However, attraction of telemedicine to patients is undeniable.

The challenge for the telecommunication community, biomedical and software engineers is to make the technology so transparent such that the physician and patient will not find it intimidating. The challenge to physicians is to acquire sufficient facility with the technology to be a competent user not subject to reliance on technical personnel.

The use of telemedicine is a fait accompli in much of the world, and it continues to have an increasing role that is deeply imbedded in our electronic practices coupled with social media. This is an opportunity for medical practice to evolve to new levels of engagement with our patients and new levels of attainment in quality of care.

Exploring the Detail of the Management Model

Most components of the model in Figure 4-2 remain invariant from enterprise to enterprise. The major elements that change are the definitions of the processes themselves, documents and technology supporting both.

The generic enterprise process model in Chapter 3 can be tailored to a specific firm, which will redefine the generic view of documents presented in Chapter 2. In turn, this will identify requirements for the technology defined in Chapter 5. Chapter 6 outlines modeling processes, analyzing dynamics of the processes with simulation, and deploying technology using object models.

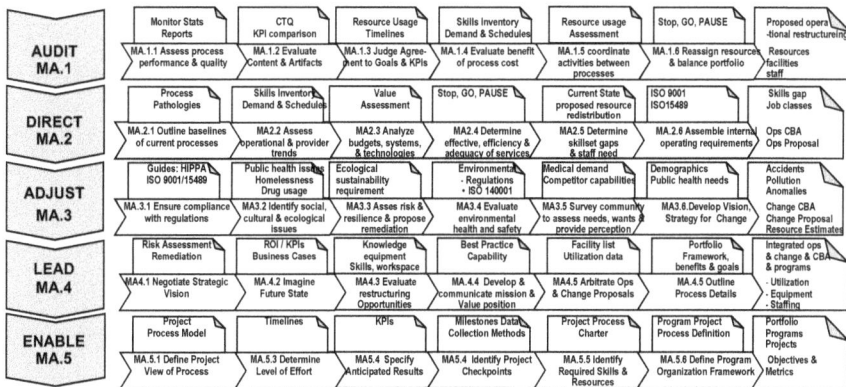

AUDIT MA.1	Monitor Stats Reports	CTQ KPI comparison	Resource Usage Timelines	Skills Inventory Demand & Schedules	Resource usage Assessment	Stop, GO, PAUSE	Proposed opera-tional restructuring
	MA.1.1 Assess process performance & quality	MA.1.2 Evaluate Content & Artifacts	MA.1.3 Judge Agreement to Goals & KPIs	MA.1.4 Evaluate benefit of process cost	MA.1.5 coordinate activities between processes	MA.1.6 Reassign resources & balance portfolio	Resources facilities staff
DIRECT MA.2	Process Pathologies	Skills Inventory Demand & Schedules	Value Assessment	Stop, GO, PAUSE	Current State proposed resource redistribution	ISO 9001 ISO15489	Skills gap Job classes
	MA.2.1 Outline baselines of current processes	MA.2.2 Assess operational & provider trends	MA.2.3 Analyze budgets, systems, & technologies	MA.2.4 Determine effective, efficiency & adequacy of services	MA.2.5 Determine skillset gaps & staff need	MA.2.6 Assemble internal operating requirements	Ops CBA Ops Proposal
ADJUST MA.3	Guides: HIPPA, ISO 9001/15489	Public health issues Homelessness Drug usage	Ecological sustainability requirement	Environmental - Regulations · ISO 140001	Medical demand Competitor capabilities	Demographics Public health needs	Accidents Pollution Anomalies
	MA.3.1 Ensure compliance with regulations	MA.3.2 Identify social, cultural & ecological issues	MA.3.3 Asses risk & resilience & propose remediation	MA.3.4 Evaluate environmental health and safety	MA.3.5 Survey community to assess needs, wants & provide perception	MA.3.6.Develop Vision, Strategy for Change	Change CBA Change Proposal Resource Estimates
LEAD MA.4	Risk Assessment Remediation	ROI / KPIs Business Cases	Knowledge equipment Skills, workspace	Best Practice Capability	Facility list Utilization data	Portfolio Framework, benefits & goals	Integrated ops & change & CBA & programs
	MA4.1 Negotiate Strategic Vision	MA.4.2 Imagine Future State	MA4.3 Evaluate restructuring Opportunities	MA.4.4 Develop & communicate mission & Value position	MA4.5 Arbitrate Ops & Change Proposals	MA.4.5 Outline Process Details	- Utilization - Equipment - Staffing
ENABLE MA.5	Project Process Model	Timelines	KPIs	Milestones Data Collection Methods	Project Process Charter	Program Project Process Definition	Portfolio Programs Projects
	MA.5.1 Define Project View of Process	MA.5.3 Determine Level of Effort	MA5.4 Specify Anticipated Results	MA5.4 Identify Project Checkpoints	MA.5.5 Identify Required Skills & Resources	MA.5.6 Define Program Organization Framework	Objectives & Metrics

Figure 4-2: *This illustrates the details of the Management Model*

The illustration shows that the Adjust functions of management are supported by the continuous improvement by Lean Six Sigma and the Simulation described in Chapter 6. The Enable function supports all of the management processes as well as all of the core processes.

Auditing provides information that indicates how to reduce time and cost and ensure quality. Time, cost and quality metrics can be continuously improved through the reduction of complexity. Consequently, the primary purpose of the auditing process must be to provide information that supports the continuous reduction of systems complexity.

The Knowledge Cycle, introduced in Chapter 2, represents the value-added activities in any process. The Knowledge Cycle defines the structure, content, and associated process to create and extend enterprise knowledge. Arbitrarily eliminating non-value-added processes may have unintended consequences because they may have been added to prevent a low probability event from causing catastrophic failure. However, in a "properly" automated process, the cycle times and variance of non-valued processes could be significantly reduced.

Auditing information quality is at the heart of productivity and governance. People need to trust the knowledge that they acquire to perform their tasks. Senior management needs to be confident that critical documents and records are authentic, reliable, accessible and have integrity. If the process is explicitly defined with a project management system and the routings effectively utilize Support Systems, then it is possible to summarize:

- Over-all process cycle time and variance,
- Value-added / non-valued added time, cost, labor ratios,
- Over-all resource utilization costs,
- Work-In-Process (WIP) costs,
- Authenticity, reliability and integrity of content.

These statistics provide the basis for making fact-based management decisions about the day-to-day operation of the process, continuous improvement, and justification for selection and deployment of systems and technology, which will innovatively improve the process.

Enterprise Metrics and Measurement

An organization must determine the metrics that are meaningful to it and define measures that reflect those metrics. Wherever possible, the actual measurements should be captured by automatically reducing both the impact on production and the burden on the worker.

How an organization defines economic value may vary from situation to situation and relies on the "Voice of the Customer." VOC involves analyzing the comments gathered in the "Define the Business" stage of Six Sigma, which is discussed in more detail in chapter 6. From these comments, the team can infer what metrics are valued.

Patient Experience	Employee Learning and Growth	Internal Process	Financial
methods and measures require answers to 3 critical questions: Who are our target patients? What is our value proposition in servicing them? What do our patients expect from our practice? Measures for the patient perspective typically are: • Overall rating of care (medical & surgical inpatients) • Overall rating of care (emergency & out-patients) • % of family physicians that receive discharge summaries • Likelihood to recommend • Employee and physician engagement & satisfaction • Community consultation measures • Transition plan measures. • Market share • Patient Retention • Patient Acquisition.	Perspective objectives and measures are the enablers of the other three perspectives. Identify the gaps between the current organizational infrastructure: • Information systems (informational capital) • Practice environment required for success (financial capital) • Grievances received and resolved prior to arbitration • % performance development plans completed/hospital policy • Vacancy rate – all nursing full time equivalents (RNs, LPNs) • Leader retention rate • Leader learning development • Staff skills (human capital) • Employee turnover • Employee satisfaction • Premium labor costs • Training and learning opportunities • Internal promotion rate • Absenteeism	Perspective identifies key processes that the practice must excel at to continue adding value for patients and practice owners. The task identifies processes that add to the value proposition and develop the best objectives and measures to track progress: • Publicly reported infection prevention and control measures • % compliance with hand hygiene: before & after patient contact • Hospital standardized mortality rate • Pressure ulcer incidents measures • Surgical safety checklist compliance • Rate of inpatient falls (harm events) • % medication reconciliation on admission. • Emergency department left without being seen • Length of stay for admitted patients • Operating room utilization • Readmission rates • Cycle-time improvement • Efficiencies in workflow • Optimization of patient-facing time	Perspective objectives and measures will tell the business owner whether the strategy execution is leading to improved bottom-line results. Typical examples include: • % alternative level of care patients • Total overtime as a % total productive hours • Nursing purchased service hours worked • Absenteeism rate • Days of cash on hand • Days in accounts receivable • Return on capital • % of billing accepted • Profitability • Revenue growth • Asset utilization

Table 4-1 Balance Score Card Metrics

Developing metrics for specific processes and projects enables companies to create a consistent set of enterprise metrics. The balance scorecard in Figure 4-3 shows a view of hospital performance by combining financial measures with operational measures of patient satisfaction, internal processes, and the organizations innovation and improvement activities – all major drivers of future performance. Sample metrics are in table 4-1.

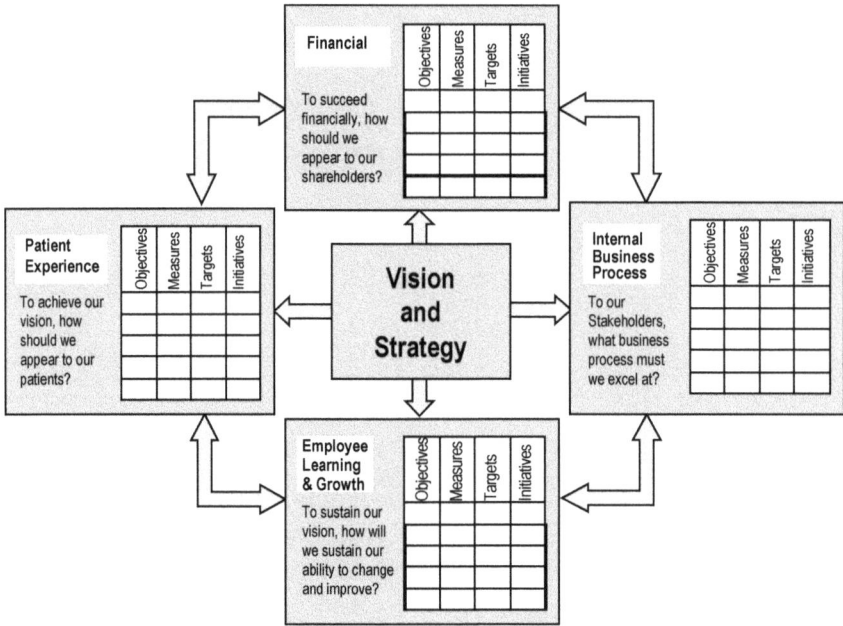

Figure 4-3: *Balanced Scorecard for Healthcare*

Program 3 Workforce Competency Projects

Problem: Medical personnel must be trained in all aspects of new interventions, rehabilitation procedures, technologies and AI to evolve toward best-practice medical care.

Purpose: Continuously improve workforce environment and competency.

Objective: Continuously evaluate collaboration progress and effective use of telemedicine.

Goal 6. Update medical staff skills to leverage changing environments and technologies:

- **Target 3.1**: Develop telemedicine proficiency.
- **Target 3.2**: Ensure the use of the latest established and approved medical procedures.
- **Target 3.3**: Enhance collaboration capabilities.

Ongoing Program Actions
- Improve the quality of telecommunication infrastructure and telemedicine capabilities.
- Continuously monitor analysis results and provide feedback on quality.
- Establish and execute a training program based on KPIs.

Key Performance Indicators	Metrics	Weight
Number of new innovations established		20%
Number of employees trained in new innovations		20%
Employee job satisfaction ratings		20%
Percentage improvement in positive patient outcomes		20%
Qualitative estimate of diagnostic correlation/causation		20%

Threats and Risks
- Proliferation of inaccurate diagnoses.
- Excessive time spent iteratively narrowing causes based on patient symptoms.

Team: Senior Manager; Computer Scientist; Process Engineer

PROJECT CHARTERS
Project 3.1: Define Collaborative Diagnostic Process
Problem: Patients with multiple symptoms often bounce between specialists for months without a clear diagnosis.

Purpose: Support primary care physicians with a team of specialists, CDS and AI to determine the cause of patient symptoms.

Objective: Use telemedicine to enable teams of specialists to assist general practitioners (GPs) in diagnosing patients.

Future State: GPs and paramedics lead specialist teams to diagnose patients more accurately and efficiently. A Clinical Decision Support (CDS) system with AI suggests potential causes, supported by telemedicine technology and high-speed telecommunications, especially in rural areas.

Actions and Deliverables
- **Culture**: Train GPs, paramedics, and diagnosticians to lead specialist teams effectively.
- **Content**: Implement a CDS system to suggest symptom causes.
- **Process**: Physicians examine patients, review lab reports, consult the CDS, and host specialist meetings.
- **Architecture**: Establish telemedicine processes and technology.
- **Infrastructure**: Provide high-speed telecommunications.

Risk: Inaccurate or misunderstood statistics result in iterative diagnoses.

Metrics: Time to correct diagnosis.

Benefits: Improved survival chances in acute cases due to earlier diagnoses.

Project 3.2: Improve Use of New Innovations

Problem: Healthcare employees misuse innovative systems.

Purpose: Train personnel to make exceptional use of new and existing innovative systems.

Objective: Train staff to ensure proficiency in use of new systems.

Future State: Staff efficiently adopt innovative systems through online training programs, reducing disruptions and maximizing system benefits.

Actions and Deliverables

- **Culture**: Train staff in the use of new or revised systems.
- **Content**: Provide online training to minimize disruptions.
- **Process**: Couple system installations with training programs.
- **Architecture**: Purchase and maintain training software.
- **Infrastructure**: Support mobile devices for training access.

Risks: Innovations may fail to deliver benefits without proper adoption.

Metrics

- Percentage of target staff trained in new systems.
- Staff ratings of training quality (Likert scale 1-5).

Benefits

- Increased staff positive attitudes toward innovative change.
- Improved ratings of technology usage and benefits.

Project 3.3: Improve Collaboration

Problem: Too many actions are taken in isolation, even when better alternatives exist.

Purpose: Train personnel to collaborate more effectively.

Objective: Use mobile devices to encourage effective knowledge transfer.

Future State: Employees actively participate in Communities of Practice (CoPs) to share knowledge and new ideas, supported by mobile apps and blogs led by subject matter experts.

Actions and Deliverables

- **Culture**: Encourage staff communication and collaboration within their specialties.
- **Content**: Develop blogs and white papers for CoPs.
- **Process**: Charter CoPs to disseminate new ideas and expertise.
- **Architecture**: Provide mobile apps for CoPs.
- **Infrastructure**: Support mobile devices for collaboration.

Risks: Failure to achieve meaningful adoption of innovations.

Metrics

- Percentage of staff trained who are CoP members.
- Staff ratings of CoPs (Likert scale 1-5).

Benefits

- Increased staff engagement with innovative changes.
- Improved technology ratings and collaborative practices.

PROGRAM 4: SUPPORT SYSTEMS

Document Technology Enables Support Systems

Implementing an enterprise support system means (re)building it, testing it, training users, deploying the system, and maintaining and improving it. Figure 5-1 illustrates the enabling support systems.

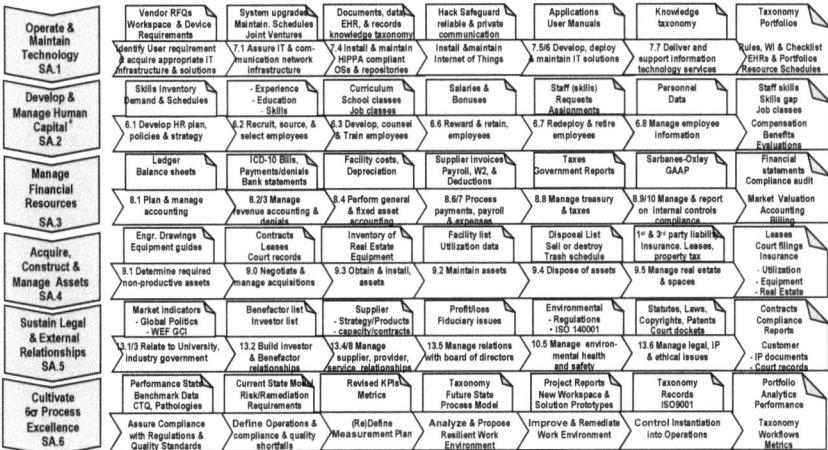

Operate & Maintain Technology SA.1	Vendor RFQs Workspace & Device Requirements	System upgrades Maintain. Schedules Joint Ventures	Documents, data EHR, & records knowledge taxonomy	Hack Safeguard reliable & private communication	Applications User Manuals	Knowledge taxonomy	Taxonomy Portfolios	
	Identify User requirement & acquire appropriate IT infrastructure & solutions	7.1 Assure IT & communication network infrastructure	7.4 Install & maintain HIPPA compliant OSs & repositories	Install &maintain Internet of Things	7.5/6 Develop, deploy & maintain IT solutions	7.7 Deliver and support information technology services	Rules, WI & Checklist EHRs & Portfolios Resource Schedules	
Develop & Manage Human Capital SA.2	Skills Inventory Demand & Schedules	- Experience - Education - Skills	Curriculum School classes Job classes	Salaries & Bonuses	Staff (skills) Requests Assignments	Personnel Data	Staff skills Skills gap Job classes	
	6.1 Develop HR plan, policies & strategy	6.2 Recruit, source, & select employees	6.3 Develop, counsel & Train employees	6.6 Reward & retain, employees	6.7 Redeploy & retire employees	6.8 Manage employee Information	Compensation Benefits Evaluations	
Manage Financial Resources SA.3	Ledger Balance sheets	ICD-10 Bills, Payments/denials Bank statements	Facility costs, Depreciation	Supplier Invoices Payroll, W2, & Deductions	Taxes Government Reports	Sarbanes-Oxley GAAP	Financial statements Compliance audit	
	8.1 Plan & manage accounting	8.2/3 Manage revenue accounting & denials	8.4 Perform general & fixed asset accounting	8.6/7 Process payments, payroll & expenses	8.8 Manage treasury & taxes	8.9/10 Manage & report on internal controls compliance	Market Valuation Accounting Billing	
Acquire, Construct & Manage Assets SA.4	Engr. Drawings Equipment guides	Contracts Leases Court records	Inventory of Real Estate Equipment	Facility list Utilization data	Disposal List Sell or destroy Trash schedule	1st & 3rd party liability Insurance. Leases, property tax	Leases Court filings Insurance	
	9.1 Determine required non-productive assets	9.0 Negotiate & manage acquisitions	9.3 Obtain & install, assets	9.2 Maintain assets	9.4 Dispose of assets	9.5 Manage real estate & spaces	- Utilization - Equipment - Real Estate	
Sustain Legal & External Relationships SA.5	Market Indicators - Global Politics - WEF GCI	Benefactor list Investor list	Supplier - Strategy/Products - capacity/contracts	Profit/loss Fiduciary issues	Environmental - Regulations - ISO 140001	Statutes, Laws, Copyrights, Patents Court dockets	Contracts Compliance Reports	
	13.1/3 Relate to University, industry government	13.2 Build investor & Benefactor relationships	13.4/8 Manage supplier, provider, service_relationships	13.5 Manage relations with board of directors	10.5 Manage environ- mental health and safety	13.6 Manage legal, IP & ethical issues	Customer - IP documents - Court records	
Cultivate 6σ Process Excellence SA.6	Performance Stats Benchmark Data CTQ, Pathologies	Current State Model Risk/Remediation Requirements	Revised KPIs Metrics	Taxonomy Future State Process Model	Project Reports New Workspace & Solution Prototypes	Taxonomy Records ISO9001	Portfolio Analytics Performance	
	Assure Compliance with Regulations & Quality Standards	Define Operations & compliance & quality shortfalls	(Re)Define Measurement Plan	Analyze & Propose Resilient Work Environment	Improve & Remediate Work Environment	Control Instantiation into Operations	Taxonomy Workflows Metrics	

Figure 5-1: The fundamental Support Systems are enabled by software

1] Operate & Maintain Technology
- Identify user requirement, acquire IT infrastructure & solutions
- Assure IT and communication network infrastructure
- Install and maintain HIPPA compliant operating system and repositories
- Install and maintain Internet of Things
- Develop, deploy and maintain IT solutions
- Deliver and support information technology services

2] Develop and Manage Human Capital
- Develop HR plan, policies and strategy

- Recruit, source, and select employees
- Develop, counsel and train employees
- Reward and retain, employees
- Redeploy and retire employees
- Manage employee information

3] Manage Financial Resources
- Plan and manage accounting
- Manage revenue accounting and denials
- Perform general and fixed asset accounting
- Process payments, payroll and expenses
- Manage treasury and taxes
- Manage and report on internal controls compliance

4] Acquire, Construct and Manage Assets
- Determine required non-productive assets
- Negotiate and manage acquisitions
- Obtain and install, assets
- Maintain assets
- Dispose of assets
- Manage real estate and spaces

5] Sustain Legal and External Relationships
- Relate to university, industry government
- Build investor and Benefactor relationships
- Manage supplier, provider, service relationships
- Manage relations with board of directors
- Manage environmental health and safety
- Manage legal, IP and ethical issues

6] Cultivate 6σ Process Excellence
- Assure Compliance with Regulations & Quality Standards
- Define Operations and compliance & quality shortfalls
- (Re)Define Measurement Plan
- Analyze and Propose Resilient Work Environment
- Improve and Remediate Work Environment
- Control Instantiation into Operations

Many healthcare organizations have spent tens of millions of dollars on hospital information technology (HIT) with no improvement in outcomes or cost. This occurs because there is no comprehensive view (model) of how processes interact across the entire hospital environment. With TDM, it becomes possible to maximize benefits from HIT. The USA Veterans Administration developed a Request for Proposal for HIT to support its 55 hospitals nation-wide. Cerner was selected to supply the system that supports the Knowledge and Document Cycles. Figure 5-2 illustrates elements of such a system. An overview of the VA RFP and PWS follows.

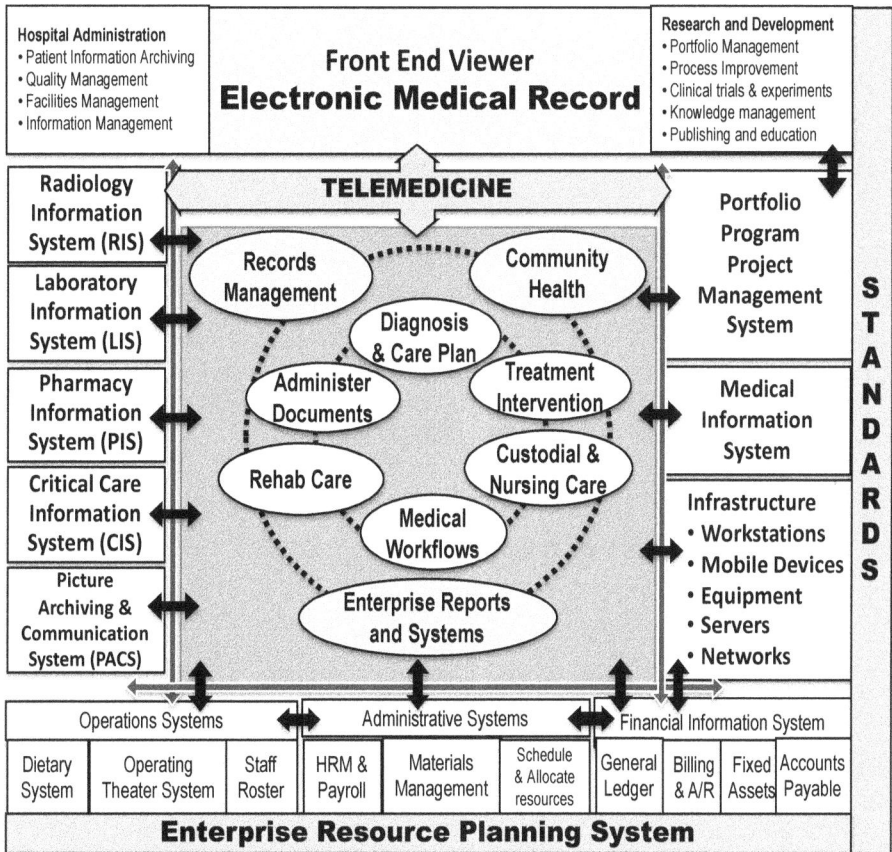

Figure 5-2: *Hospital Information Systems*

In May 2018, the U.S. Department of Veterans Affairs (VA) awarded a contract to Cerner Corporation to modernize its Electronic Health Record (EHR) system. The primary objective was to ensure interoperability between the VA and Department of Defense (DoD) health systems, allowing for seamless sharing of patient data among VA, DoD, and community healthcare providers.

The VA's decision to select Cerner was influenced by the DoD's prior adoption of Cerner's EHR system, known as MHS GENESIS. By aligning with the same platform, the VA aimed to eliminate the challenges associated with disparate systems and ensure a unified approach to veteran healthcare records. The contract included system configuration, data migration from existing systems and technology, user training, and ongoing support to ensure system's successful implementation and sustainability.

The Performance Work Statement (PWS) associated with the Veterans Affairs (VA) Request for Proposal (RFP) for the Cerner Electronic Health Record (EHR) modernization outlines the comprehensive requirements for implementing an interoperable and scalable health information system tailored to the needs of the VA. Below is a summary of its key elements:

1. Scope of Work

The PWS specifies the procurement, configuration, deployment, and maintenance of a Commercial Off-The-Shelf (COTS) EHR solution. It requires full interoperability with:

- The Department of Defense (DoD) EHR system.
- Community healthcare providers.
- Existing VA systems and workflows.
- The objective is to provide a unified and seamless health record system for veterans across all VA facilities.

2. System Requirements

- Functional Specifications:
    - Comprehensive patient record management for inpatient, outpatient, and specialized care.
    - Integration with laboratory, pharmacy, imaging, and other clinical modules.

- Support for telehealth services and mobile devices.
- Technical Specifications:
    - Compliance with federal IT standards, including HIPAA and NIST security frameworks.
    - Scalability to accommodate millions of veteran records.
    - High availability, redundancy, and disaster recovery capabilities.

3. Data Migration and Integration
- Legacy System Migration:
    - Transition of data from VISTA (Veterans Health Information. Systems and Technology Architecture) to the new EHR.
    - Validation and verification to ensure data accuracy and integrity.
- Interoperability Requirements:
    - Real-time data exchange with DoD's MHS GENESIS.
    - APIs for integration with external healthcare providers and systems.

4. Training and Change Management
- Training Program:
    - Comprehensive training for healthcare providers, IT staff, and administrative users.
    - Multi-tiered training approach: basic, advanced, and role-specific modules.
- Change Management:
    - Strategies to ease the transition for stakeholders and end-users.
    - Continuous feedback mechanisms to refine system usability.

5. Deployment Strategy
- Phased Rollout:
    - Implementation across all VA medical facilities in planned waves.
    - Priority given to high-impact regions for initial deployment.
- Pilot Testing:
    - Testing in controlled environments to identify and mitigate issues.
    - User acceptance testing (UAT) before full-scale implementation.

6. Performance Metrics
- Key Performance Indicators (KPIs):
    - System uptime and responsiveness.
    - Reduction in patient record errors.

- Improvements in care delivery metrics, such as appointment scheduling times.
- Reporting: Monthly performance reviews with detailed system analytics.

7. Ongoing Support and Maintenance
- Technical Support:
  - 24/7 helpdesk services for system users.
  - Periodic updates and patches to address vulnerabilities and enhance features.
- System Monitoring:
  - Automated tools for monitoring system performance and user activity.
  - Proactive measures to prevent outages or data breaches.

8. Compliance and Security
- Adherence to VA and DoD security protocols.
- Integration of audit trails for accountability and transparency.
- Regular compliance reviews and updates to address evolving regulations.

9. Cost and Value Optimization
- Efficient use of resources to minimize costs without compromising functionality.
- Use of cloud-based services where applicable to reduce infrastructure requirements.
- Periodic reviews to ensure alignment with budget and timelines.

This detailed PWS forms the backbone of the VA's strategy to modernize its EHR system while ensuring interoperability, security, and enhanced healthcare delivery for veterans.

Overview of ERP in Healthcare

Enterprise Resource Planning (ERP) systems are centralized software platforms designed to streamline operations, improve efficiency, and reduce costs. In healthcare, these systems integrate various functions—ranging from patient records to financial management—into a unified platform, enabling better decision-making and enhanced patient care.

Core Features of Healthcare ERP Systems

1. Real-Time Information: Access to up-to-date data for operational transparency.

2. Automation: Streamlines workflows, reduces errors, and eliminates redundant data entry.

3. Centralized Data Management: Ensures all departments can share and access critical information seamlessly.

4. Decision Support: Provides analytics and reporting tools to guide organizational strategies.

5. Efficiency Boost: Minimizes redundancies and fosters cross-department collaboration.

6. Scalability: Adapts to organizational growth and evolving needs.

7. Security: Protects sensitive data through robust security measures.

8. Integration Capabilities: Connects with external systems via APIs or connectors.

9. Cloud-Based Flexibility: Offers reduced infrastructure costs and simplified maintenance.

10. Customizability: Tailored solutions for specific healthcare workflows.

Benefits of ERP in Healthcare

1. Financial Management: Automation of budgeting, forecasting, and expense tracking.

2. Supply Chain Optimization: Efficient inventory and procurement management.

3. HR Management: Streamlines onboarding, training, and performance tracking.

4. Operational Efficiency: Enhances communication across departments.

5. Regulatory Compliance: Ensures adherence to industry and federal standards.

6. Patient Care Improvements: Enables better diagnostics and treatment planning.

7. Cost Savings: Consolidates systems and standardizes processes.

8. Data Analytics: Offers insights for strategic decision-making.

9. Cloud Computing: Enables secure, scalable, and mobile-friendly operations.

Types of ERP Systems
1. Cloud-Based ERP: Accessible from anywhere, with features like automatic updates and scalability.
2. On-Premises ERP: Installed locally for firms requiring complete control.
3. Hybrid ERP: Combines the benefits of cloud and on-premises systems for flexibility and resilience.

Applications of ERP in Healthcare
- Financial Management: Centralized tracking and auditing of transactions.
- HR Management: Effective workforce planning and compliance.
- Materials Management: Optimizes inventory and vendor relations.
- Patient Administration: Streamlines processes like billing, admissions, and records management.
- Workflow Optimization: Automates clinical and administrative tasks.

Healthcare ERP systems are transformative tools that optimize hospital operations and enhance patient care. Despite implementation challenges, working with experienced service providers ensures a smooth transition. This guide offers a comprehensive foundation for understanding how ERP systems like EPIC and Cerner can be deployed to modernize healthcare operations effectively.

ERP systems for managing purchasing, inventories and the supply chain can be much more extensive and complex for manufacturing. Managing patients as portfolios of projects makes managing HRM more complex in healthcare and billing is guided by 144,000 WHO ICD-10 codes.

Home Health Technology

Chapter 3 asserted the use of telemedicine and other devices for the elderly in the home as well as in nursing homes and all adult-living facilities may be superior to office visits in terms of hospitalizations, complications, emergency visits, and quality of life for rehabilitation after stroke, diabetes, hypertension, pain, congestive heart failure, and cancer care.

Telemedicine interventions in home health are provided around the clock. Furthermore, the home health nurse alone when confronted by a worrisome change can only order transfer to definitive diagnosis and care or communicate by phone with the managing physician. Instead, telemedicine as an augmentation to the physical visit, can be used by nurses to transfer images to evaluate skin lesions or gait, to discuss telemetry data, and receive new instructions which otherwise would only be possible after a visit by the patient to the physician's office. Another use of telemedicine in home healthcare is the critical support of home caregivers who are subject to exhaustion, terrible stress, and a strong urge at times to give up and send the house-bound patient to a facility. Telemedicine creates a virtual team that can include the home caregiver and dispel the sense of isolation. Home is best as long as possible. The alternative of travel to a fixed health facility is tedious, labor intensive, painful, and expensive.

Simple monitoring devices can assess gait, pace, activity in general, and adherence to a medical regimen. Sleep, falls, body functions, blood pressure, pulse, oxygen saturation and weight monitoring can be done with non-invasive sensors, and the data can be transferred wirelessly to a computer for transmission to a health management office. The management site can look for alerts and trends with a response that is anywhere from a call to a summon of emergency personnel to the home, to changing medication with a message back to the patient.

Inexpensive sensors, either passive or interactive, can capture the essence of a health situation at home and the managing physician can provide immediate care available only otherwise in the hospital or office. Instead of a visit on demand from time to time or regularly every month, surveillance can inform the physician about the situation and allow timely and effective intervention. A smart home with sensors and alerts can assess the environment for such subtleties as a running tub, temperature of the water, age of materials in the refrigerator, consumption of food, water, and medications as well as the urgent situations indicated by the presence of smoke, carbon monoxide, or excess heat. Mobile phones can provide information support and alerts to the home bound.

Medical apps for smartphones can be incorporated into comprehensive home health plans by a managing physician with patient consent. Smart-phone programs are excellent for behavior modification for weight, diet, smoking cessation, medication, alcohol abuse, and exercise. Increasingly, medical practices are using social media to enrich medical practice through enhanced communication and reminders to reinforce a regimen.

Cohesion and awareness of diagnostic complexity is not enough to make an organization operationally adaptive. Effective R&D is critical in insuring that a healthcare organization will continue to improve as patient census changes, interventions evolve, and new medications and technologies become available. An R&D strategy along with a hospital systems process model must be clearly and explicitly defined along with benefits, which are expected to accrue from a well-run portfolio of programs and their associated projects. To achieve this objective, the standard that supports this activity is the Project Management Institute's (PMI) standards for portfolio program and project management.

Portfolio, Program and Project Framework

PMI's standards are impressive, however, lack of recursion from portfolio to program to project is unfortunate because in their current form "roll-ups" are not possible. We have reworked the standards so that at a high-level view they are recursive – they roll-up visually - where all three levels in the hierarchy are defined by the process in Figure 5-3.

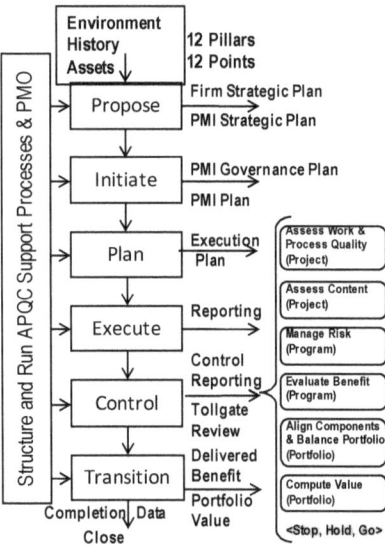

PMI's standards for portfolio, program, and project management are a key component in the foundation for creating innovation through R&D processes as part of managing organizational complexity. Strategy is restricted to contain only portfolios, portfolios to contain only programs and programs to contain only projects. Also, the concept of a project is expanded to be 'called' repeatedly and concurrently. This allows the use of the standard everywhere in the organization.

Figure 5-3: Portfolio / Project Management

Portfolios are integral to an organization's strategic plan and its governance. Programs guide the execution of projects, which make up all processes including R&D. Control reporting and tollgate reviews allow the portfolio and program sponsors to evaluate whether the proposed benefits are or will be realized. These reviews decide whether to stop, hold, or go.

In this context, we consider an organization to be made up of various segments of profound knowledge from Deming's book, The New Economics, which cannot be separated. Each segment interacts with the others as follows:

- Appreciation for the System: Network components that work together.
- Knowledge of Variation: If a process is not in a state of statistical control, cost, performance, quality and quantity are not predictable.
- Psychology: Nurture and preserve positive innate attributes of people.
- Theory of Knowledge: (discussed earlier).

This leads us to the question of what portfolio elements and programs do tollgate reviews use to assess project value, particularly where patients are a Portfolio of programs. The general vision is new, faster, better and/or cheaper now and in future operations.

A portfolio contains a balanced scorecard and key performance indicators (KPI), that allow portfolio and program sponsors to assess progress. This includes patient flow to wellness, better utilization of critical equipment, resource and facilities, and improved staff competencies. Successful delivery of R&D projects should increase the R&D portfolio value and an organization's economic value-added (EVA).

Hypothetical R & D Portfolio
Ensuring innovation also requires the establishment of a portfolio for R&D projects because of the need for an Organizational Strategic Plan:

- Vision: New, faster, better, cheaper now and later
- Mission: Profitable, adaptive and competitive
- Value: Organizational KPIs to improve EVA
- R&D portfolio contains programs with KPIs
- Delight the (patient) client with quality outcomes
- Reduce time-to-complete (patient) client solutions
- Provide exceptional governance
- Assure quality management of records
- Improve operational performance (cheaper/better)
- Increase number of (patients) customers

- Improve individual competency and capability
- Improve collaboration / workgroup performance
- Accelerate knowledge flow to patient value
- Improve access to and quality of records (EHR)

Successful delivery of R&D programs increases R&D portfolio value and organizational EVA leading to improved (patient) customer outcomes too.

Portfolio Management

Portfolio management is about value and project management is about cost control and delivery. Both are essential for innovation. A portfolio rolls up component projects into various programs within the portfolio. Portfolio management informs program management with strategies and objectives that are clear and advantageous with a clear definition of desired outcomes. To make portfolio management work, it must employ new systems and processes, portals that provide shared access to data and documents, and visualization tools to support decision-making.

Program 4 Projects for Support Systems

Problem: Promote population health while delivering best-practice healthcare and long-term care.

Purpose: Leverage support systems and technology to configure system support for all medical entities in the region.

Objective: Continuously evaluate and improve wellness outcomes for chronically ill patients to enhance quality of life for those in long-term care.

Goal 7: Minimize resource costs while ensuring availability and capability of facilities and positive patient outcomes:

- **Target 4.1**: Right-size staff for any given patient population census.
- **Target 4.2**: Minimize inventories while ensuring adequate supplies are always available.
- **Target 4.3**: Optimize facility utilization.

Program Scope

- **In Scope**: Population within the health system region.
- **Out of Scope**: Restricted to people in medical facilities.

Ongoing Program Actions

- Monitor and promote wellness within the community.
- Evaluate staff performance and utilization.
- Assess the use and maintenance of disposable products.
- Monitor and evaluate facility utilization and maintenance.

Key Performance Indicators	Metrics	Weight
Staff utilization percentage		30%
Number of patients completing programs		30%
Inventory turns		20%
Facility utilization percentage		20%

Threats and Risks

- Insufficient patient numbers or ineffective interventions may fail to improve quality of life.
- Poorly configured systems lead to wasted time, money, and resources.

Team: Project Manager; Accountant; Lawyer; HRM and IT Specialists

PROJECT CHARTERS

Project 4.1: (Re)Configure EHR system to consolidate patient records

Problem: Patient records are often disjointed, lost, or improperly maintained.

Purpose: Maintain comprehensive patient medical histories across providers.

Objective: Implement or reconfigure an EHR system with a HIPAA-compliant repository to retain patient records.

Actions and Deliverables

- **Culture**: Train medical staff to use the EHR system effectively.
- **Content**: Ensure all patient information, procedures, and results are available online including statistics of patient flow.
- **Process**: Facilitate system-wide interaction among medical personnel during flow to wellness aided by simulation.
- **Architecture**: Deployed EHR and CDS software.
- **Infrastructure**: Provide mobile device access to the software.

Risks: Incomplete or inaccurate records could lead to incorrect diagnoses.

Metrics

- Percentage of ISO 15489-compliant records.
- Percent of interoperable records across medical facilities in the region.

Benefits

- Improved understanding of patient history for better diagnostics.
- Enhanced AI-driven CDS accuracy using anonymous records.
- Automated administrative tasks.

Project 4.2: Configure ERP and CDS to optimize delivery of care

Problem: Patients face delays when staff, resources, and facilities are unavailable and path to wellness is not defined.

Purpose: Ensure a continuous flow of patients to wellness through a hospital system while optimizing resources and use of equipment and facilities.

Objective: Effectively use ERP and CDS software to schedule patient procedures, schedule critical staff, equipment, facilities and resources.

Actions and Deliverables

- **Culture**: Train medical personnel in ERP, CDS and AI use.

- **Content**: Provide online access to staff and resource usage statistics.
- **Process**: Coordinate administrative of patient transitions.
- **Architecture**: Deploy and/or reconfigure ERP and CDS software.
- **Infrastructure**: Provide mobile device access to the system.
- **Risk:** Incomplete or inaccurate statistics lead to inefficiencies.

Metrics

• Percentage of beds filled.	• Profit margins.
• Percent OR room usage.	• Inventory turns.
• Cost of disposables.	• Iterations to correct diagnosis
• Percentage rejected bills.	• Time to diagnosis

Benefits
- Improved patient flow and resource management.
- Enhanced AI-driven CDS accuracy using anonymous records.
- Automated administrative processes.
- Faster treatment of life-threatening conditions.
- Reduced delays in diagnosis and treatment.

Project 4.3: Install visualization capability

Problem: Patients in remote, emergency, or in-home settings often lack adequate care and information to manage daily activities.

Purpose: Provide high-quality visual telecommunication anytime, anywhere.

Objective: Provide telemedicine to remote areas and performance dashboard for managers.

Actions and Deliverables
- **Culture**: Train paramedics to use a virtual ER
- **Content**: Ensure all required medical and operations data is accessible from portable and big screen devices
- **Process**: Facilitate visual interaction with medical systems.
- **Architecture**: Deployed telecommunication and display capability.
- **Infrastructure**: Assure mobile device access to all hospital systems.

Metrics
- Percent increase in patients treated outside hospitals using telemedicine.
- Faster response to operational requirements

Benefits
- Improved care for remote and outpatient populations.
- Enhanced access to specialists in geographically dispersed areas.
- Improved operational management.
- Enhanced decision-making based on statistics rather than just intuition.

6

An Introduction to Change

Organizations are dynamic, and TDM is a flexible, powerful method for driving enterprise transformation. To guide change RDM focuses on:

- Ensuring knowledge and records are accessible when needed (Axiom 1).
- Supporting knowledge flow through processes and documenting value creation (Axiom 2).
- Building models to assess the current state and explore "what-if" scenarios (Axiom 2).
- Educating individuals in critical skills and rewarding continuous learning (Axiom 3).
- Leveraging support systems and network infrastructure (Axiom 4).
- Automating knowledge flow and integrating software applications using advanced technology (Axiom 4).

'TDM I' was published in 1999, one year before Thomas Pyzdek published the first edition of the 6σ Handbook. Thomas Pyzdek and Paul Keller 720 page Six Sigma Handbook 2023 6th edition represents a robust and tested methodology, but TDM does a better job of defining "Policy."

Lean 6σ process: DMAIC (Define/Measure>Analyze>Improve>Control). emphasizes the importance of quality, measurement and efficiency because they have all grown out of Deming's manufacturing methodology.

This chapter articulates TDM's perspective that underpins an effective environment for health and elder care. This approach is predicated on a convergence of existing and highly regarded strategies for management and information flow with mechanisms and culture driving modes of communication and visualization. Technical innovation informs a general understanding of what is possible and identifies evolving systems predicated on best practice technological infrastructure and methodologies.

With respect to healthcare, expectations are arising from a general awareness of advances in technology and personal experience:
- Views on medical data accessibility and ownership
- Expectations regarding collaborative diagnosis through contemporary modes of communication and visualization
- Timely diagnosis to reduce patient anxiety through delay
- Expedient remediation of illness and rehabilitation
- Reduced costs to both patient and society

TDM is built on content flow and disposition of documents, records and knowledge flow to value and collects these methods into a unified approach to change. Integral to this approach identified in previous chapters was ISO 15489, APQC process framework, VSM, Carnegie Mellon's People CMM, Porter's Integrated Practice Unit, Lynn's Medicaring model, Balanced Scorecard, and PMI's portfolio, program and project management.

LEAN Six Sigma (6σ) is used to identify and implement local efficiencies that can be monitored from higher organizational levels. Lean 6σ is a methodology to control operations, resulting in high quality products. Its advocates require senior managers to set policy, goals and objectives that direct change projects to make the enterprise "better." It proposes taking baby steps to successful measurable conclusions.

However, management cannot set goals to get somewhere without knowing where they are? LEAN 6σ is focused on defining a project portfolio and successfully completing it, not on outlining the portfolio structure.

To set policy, goals and objectives to transform the firm, managers must: 1] know how knowledge flows to value EVERYWHERE, 2] define POLICY and outline a portfolio to leverage EXISTING skills, operations and technology better, then use Lean 6σ to continuously improve the firm with assurance that "baby step" projects go in the intended direction.

Chapter 6 describes at three perspectives to improve a firm's effectiveness, efficiency and profitability: TDM, Lean 6σ and CSI's 12 Point Plan.

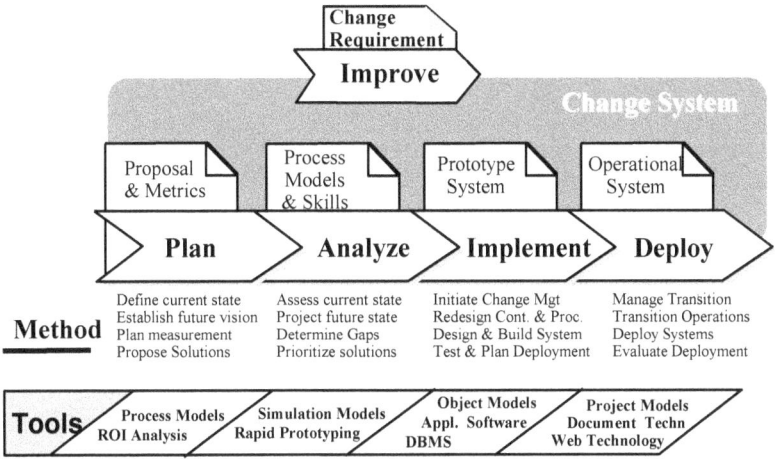

Figure 6-1: *Change process steps are plan, analyze, implement and deploy.*

The Core Process Model for Change in Enterprise

Figure 6-1 illustrates change in The Document Method for changing business processes in these four steps:

Plan	with an enterprise document strategy that identifies the current state and proposes a future vision and metrics with an approach to
Analyze	by synchronizing document flow as output of business processes that provide information to
Implement	rapidly prototyped document systems that continuously eliminate bottlenecks to
Deploy	a business environment for workgroups to run core processes with knowledge based value-added documents.

For those who are committed to a specific process change, continuous improvement or total quality management methodology like Six Sigma or Lean, establishing knowledge flow to value must be the first project. Once management knows how it creates value from its knowledge, it can set policy, goals, objectives, priorities, a portfolio of programs and a balanced scorecard so that a path forward can be defined in project plans. Because LEAN 6σ has become ubiquitous, its relationship to TDM follows.

Plan (6σ Define/Measure)

Senior management plays a key role in supporting innovation that springs from the factual base of TDM. Accordingly, management must set a strategic direction and define priorities. Planning must understand the current state, develop a vision that embraces a Document Strategy, identify gaps and select measures to close gaps. Planning employs elements defined by methods in Chapter 2, to capture and communicate knowledge in a document architecture. Successfully implemented, the document architecture will ensure critical knowledge about a process is recorded.

Analyze

Analyze defines and uses a high-level core process model of document flow, like the generic process model outlined in Chapter 3 to communicate and identify major bottlenecks. It is not appropriate to initiate a time-based simulation until results of initial iterations provide a project view of process with documents as milestones is adopted and supported by the technology in Chapter 5. Initially an "almost AS IS" view of the organization is developed to determine what improvements and innovations can be accomplished immediately. This includes defining requirements for the document technology that must be installed to reduce process bottlenecks.

Implement (6σ Improve)

Implement prototypes with technology described in Chapter 5 to make exceptional use of existing and commercial technology. This implementation assures that knowledge is accessible, and its use is recorded everywhere in the enterprise. Methods for Axiom 4 provide information to assemble and make exceptional use of new technology.

Deploy (6σ Control)

The concept of viable systems is discussed in Chapter 4, *Managing the Enterprise*. A viable system defines the elements of an empowered business process. Methods for Axiom 3 provide information to control deploying change:

- Understand management as a process -- lead, improve, direct, enable.
- Derive facts to manage using transaction knowledge from monitoring.
- Install metrics to define, audit and benchmark process performance.
- Teach the methods described below in a continuous learning program.

Knowledge flow to value in an organization is significantly impacted by its employees' ability to collaborate. Improving their ability to collaborate can be guided by the 12 Point Plan for Effective Collaboration (developed by CSI, Pty Ltd). The 12-points are a diagnostic tool and transition method to create an appropriate level of innovation readiness that accelerates knowledge flow to value.

Precedence to consider is the Australian Government's use as guidance material for implementing the government's R&D Tax Incentive. The 12 points framework provided a back-drop to the guidelines, learning and development, and the evaluation of R&D governance and knowledge management capabilities of companies claiming the tax incentive.

The 12 points assess organizational complexity by enumerating issues associated with how firms manage A) basic requirements, B) efficiency and C) innovation, which correspond to the 12 pillars of WEF GCI. (www.weforum.org/reports/the-global-competitveness-report-2018).

A. Basic Requirements

- Strategy and scope: (vision and mission) establishes the organization's knowledge flow to customer value and assures its financial viability.
- Guiding Principles: balance innovative change and operational excellence based on knowledge and skills flowing to customer value.
- Capability and competencies: emphasize the ways people collaborate and leverage and improve each other's skills and knowledge.
- Workspaces: empower collaborative workgroups and specific work functions of individuals.

B. Efficiency Enhancers

- Planning: arbitrates between marketing innovation and operations to budget resources to accelerate knowledge flow to products or services.
- Position: examines the political, socio-economic, technological factors that influence position, customer needs, staff competencies, resources.
- Training/Recruitment: identify gaps in people's knowledge, capability and competence to bridge those gaps with mentors and training.
- Competitiveness/collaborative workgroups: improve competencies, work practices, technology to excel at cost, quality, and/or innovation.

- Work practices and measurement: establish workflows to examine and measure ways teams achieve results, and how they collaborate, innovate, share and acquire new knowledge.
- IT platforms and virtual environments are central to a collaborative, integrated business strategy. Visualization must be employed to increase effectiveness of communication over distance.

C. Innovation

- Standards and knowledge management: guide the capture, management and flow of knowledge & know-how as competitive advantage assets.
- Learning and expertise networks: identify and catalogue biographies of trusted experts to use them effectively; mentor and document lessons learned to record experiential knowledge.

To reduce the cost of healthcare within a community, state or nation, it is necessary to consider the full gamut of collaborative possibilities from the patient environment both inside and outside the hospital, especially when the elderly are in a frail state. Health, home and hygiene are integrated elements of the total system. The 12 points methodology creates a healthcare environment where value can be explicitly defined in a variety of ways: diagnosis, intervention, home support, rehab and medication.

Using Analysis

Examining knowledge flow to customer value is critical in assessing the current state. Critical enterprise documents are identified and assigned lifecycles that trace their transition from ad-hoc documents through validated revisions to records.

Explicit definition of business is derived from methods of Axiom 1-3. Axiom 1 assures that the purpose of documents is understood and classified. Axiom 2 defines processes as projects with documents as milestones. Axiom 3 focuses on the competencies required to support knowledge flow through process to create value for the customer.

The activities necessary to create, validate and manage lifecycles of critical documents are identified. From this process, document and process pathologies and lack of competence are postulated.

Define the Future State

The first step in transitioning to the future state is to reduce current state process pathologies. They are found by asking questions such as, does one part of the organization redo the work of another? Is the knowledge required available? Documents may be misfiled (electronic or paper), or in an unusable format (wrong file format, foreign language).

Transitioning to a future state vision improves products, makes documents more comprehensible, eliminates process bottlenecks and unnecessary documents and improves governance and compliance. In the first step, an "almost" current state also represents the future state where the changes are made to technology, skills, collaborative methods and infrastructure to ensure that the organization becomes more effective, efficient and adaptive.

Determine Gaps and Weaknesses

Once the knowledge flow to value is clearly understood and more detail is built around the future state, critical gaps and weaknesses will be illuminated. At this point, the analysis team must consider problem/solution alternatives and prioritize them based on potential ROI, level of difficulty and resources required, risk mitigation and making exceptional use of legacy and new commercial systems. Solutions will include document, process, competency and system changes for each problem.

Consider Solutions

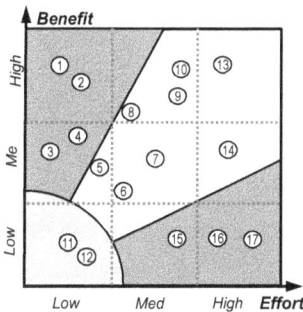

Figure 6-2: Benefit vs, Effort

Problem/solution alternatives must then be defined as projects. **Effort** is based on the project plans, resource requirements, project duration, risk, capital investment and new skills and system costs. **Benefit** of each project with respect to impact on revenue, customer satisfaction, potential to leverage existing systems and fit with a future state vision must be judged. Figure 6-2 plots Benefit vs. Effort.

Solutions are crafted in terms of Business Cases where the value of culture, content, process and system changes are described and quantified.

Culture makes information meaningful, by interpreting people's experience and helping them decide how to act. In this sense, knowledge is actionable information. E.g., if an employee is an experienced tool and die maker, he can build a product by interpreting an assembly drawing.

Content design is focused on presenting information to invoke desirable behaviors in the information consumer (e.g., filling out forms properly).

Process represents tasks people perform to create value for their customers. Once knowledge and content objects that deliver value are identified, it is possible to redefine the process to permit monitoring, measurement and acceleration of knowledge flow to value and compute ROI.

Systems ensure that knowledge is optimally accessible, managed and archived using global information networks, collaboration technologies and the web. They are key to building knowledge environments that improve a corporation's ability to compete on its knowledge.

Models and Modeling

For each current state core process map the following: Supplier -> Inputs -> Process (Sub-Tasks, Competencies, Systems) -> Outputs -> Customers. Whether acquired through reading, interviews, observations or workshops, questions to be answered for each critical area are identified in Table 6-1.

Measures	Constraints	Document Lifecycle
Finance? Customer? Learning? Operations? Systems? Support? Cycle time? Cost? Quality?	What starts the process? Document? Question? Problem? What guides & constrains the work? Policy? Budget? Procedure? Drawing? Menu? Work Instruction? Etc?	Create – Amend – Publish – Store – Archive – Destroy How many people edit, read, manage documents? Where? When? Policies? IT? What security is required?
Inputs What does the process use? consume? Materials? Documents? Expert advice?	**Process** What is the department, Process or Function? How is it measured? What is the Parent process? What are the sub-tasks?	**Outputs** What are the deliverables? Product Components? Documents? Advice? Is this a component of an assembled output? Who is & what delights customers?
Sub tasks What are the answers to these questions for sub-tasks? How are sub-tasks broken down? Skill? Work volume? Natural Checkpoints? Responsibilities/turf? Random? Ad-hoc?	**Mechanisms** Who does the work? Groups? Vendors? How many? How much? What competencies & skills? What systems are used? How are documents stored? How do people work? Adversarial? Independent? Collaborative? Physical Proximity of people? Means of communication?	**Future State** How can information be reused? How can documents/ knowledge be shared? Be controlled? approvals be accelerated? How can existing systems improve management of knowledge? How can consistent, reliable access to documents/ knowledge be provided from anywhere?

Table 6-1: Questions for Analysis of Current and Future States

Table 6-2 shows TDM healthcare model process detail.

1.0 Market	3.3 Manage orders
1.1 Understand patients, markets, & capabilities	3.4 Analyze usage
1.2 Define community marketing strategy	3.5 (Re)define quality processes
1.3 Coordinate with social programs	**4.0 Deliver**
1.4 Diagnose Participants & Plan Care	4.1 Administer In-patient records & documents
1.5 Solicit sources of revenue	4.2 Diagnose In-patient & Plan Care
2.0 Develop	4.3 Provide In-patient Intervention
2.1 Configure portfolio	4.4 Provide In-patient Therapy
2.2 Set up Project Management Office	4.5 Provide In-patient Custodial Care
2.3 Oversee programs	**5.0 Maintain**
2.4 Test market for new/revised services	5.1 Administer Out-patient records & documents
3.0 Purchase	5.2 Diagnose Out-patient & Plan Care
3.1 Define purchasing strategy	5.3 Provide Out-patient Intervention
3.2 Qualify & select suppliers	5.4 Provide Out-patient Therapy
	5.5 Provide Out-patient Custodial Care

Table 6-2: TDM / Process Detail

Figure 6-3 shows a network of all the models.

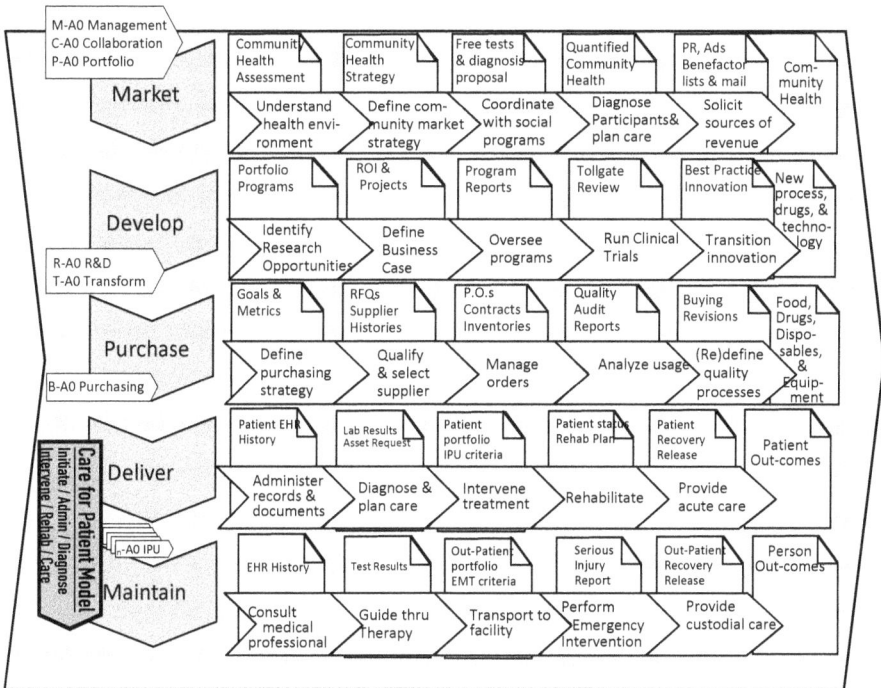

Figure 6-3: A0 Run Health System

A0 Run Health System (Introduction), **H-A0 Healthcare** (Chapter 3), **M-A0 Management** (Chapter 4), **S-A0 Support** (Chapter 5), were presented together in the Introduction after Figure 1-2.

Other Models in the TDM III Methodology

T-A0 Transform is the change process defined by this chapter.

C-A0 Collaboration is well established and has been used in many industries; it guides best practice for medical personnel who must collaborate in physical and virtual situations: e.g., a GP leads a team of specialists to diagnose and plan an intervention and rehab program for a patient; a patient is examined by a physician's assistant in a rural health center who telecommunicates with a physician in a major health center; a paramedic at an emergency site telecommunicates with a hospital ER.

E-A0 EMS was derived from an analysis of rural healthcare and emergency medical services; best practice requires telemedicine.

I_n-A0 IPU may require a separate process model for each of the 16 complex care areas listed in chapter 3. A major hospital must determine how to minimize its number of IPU models.

A-A0 Tollgate defines how portfolio, programs and projects must be audited as defined by the PMI's Book of Knowledge.

B-A0 Purchase (Buy) supports 3. Purchase; it is well established and has been used in many industries including healthcare equipment and pharmaceutical manufacturing.

R-A0 R&D supports **Develop**; it is well established with its use in many industries including a project to support the Australian government's program that allows companies to receive tax concessions for doing innovative research. The program outlines a model for defining a portfolio of R&D projects and defines how they will be audited by Tollgate Review.

P-A0 Portfolio is essentially defined by PMI's Book of Knowledge, but has been redefined so that its processes are recursive across projects, programs and portfolios.

Implement involves designing and prototyping the document delivery business environment. Integrating existing tools and commercially available software minimizes costs of systems development. The prototype is released to users to beta test the system in an environment that includes the future state content, process and competency changes. Revisions to all areas are made as necessary in anticipation of deployment.

Initiate Change Management

A transition plan and communication program define how the production system is deployed. It provides the framework for communication to develop the prototype, establish the Program Management Office (PMO) and deploy the production system. Marketing and business justification toward specific departments is based on a business case unique to a department. Departments will share the results of the ongoing studies to build a common knowledge base on performed studies and the results.

Redesign Content and Processes

Installing and testing support systems to insure β systems viability involves change in culture, content, and process.

- Identify critical knowledge that delivers value to the customer.
- Define an enterprise knowledge taxonomy with metadata and keywords to assure accessibility.
- Structure document templates for comprehensibility to capture critical knowledge content.
- Monitor document reuse, age, keyword and metadata usage and authentication.
- Model core processes to identify critical document links and synergies.
- Define a project view of process with document milestones.
- Instantiate the process with workflow and monitor knowledge.

Design and Configure Systems

Installing and testing support systems may require a significant work effort involved in moving data and documents to a newly reconfigured repository. In addition to integrating existing technology, there is commercially available software described in Chapter 5.

The deployment process step must minimize the risk of changing processes. New technology is used to explicitly define a process so that its variation can be calculated and reduced.

Establish a PMO

Program Management Office (PMO) submits a monthly activity report to the senior manager responsible for the Program Office and a quarterly employee electronic newsletter. This report will include the status of all projects. PMO will continuously promote project benefits and progress with planned road shows and conferences. All five programs and their projects report to the PMO.

Manage Transition

Successful deployment depends on deploying methodology and technology and understanding all of the dimensions in the business environment.

- Knowledge must be accessible and comprehensible; its flow to value must be quantified and measured.
- Processes must be explicitly defined, with documents as milestones of a project view of process.
- People must comprehend that the desired state will improve the company's ability to compete on knowledge. Managers must be held accountable to manage, monitor, measure and improve process.
- Systems integrated with infrastructure require adequate network infrastructure, capacity, security and availability and installation and administration of a full set of applications,
- Financial. Functional elements must be scalable, and cost effectively support business requirements.
- The future state is continually re-evaluated as technology, methodology and skills evolve.

Transition Operations

Specify and deploy a program to create an operational vision of what it means to "compete on knowledge" as an employee's future state:

- A marketing campaign to persuade staff knowledge access is critical,
- Facilitate internal and external communities to determine best practice.
- Educate employees in future state best practices.
- Specify methods for process, content, and cultural change.
- Create a collaboration group of thought leaders in diverse business.
- Deploy a support to purchase, install, maintain and manage technology.

Deploy Systems in Business Environments

- Deploy a business workgroup environment that satisfies the future state recommendations.
- Deploy business cases satisfying business ROE.
- Deploy a set of services based on business case profiles.
- Migrate legacy systems.
- Deploy the selected technology.

TDM and Lean Six Sigma (6σ)

TDM would consider replacing 'Implement' and 'Deploy' with an approach based on 6σ DMAIC. 6σ is illustrated in Figure 6-4. Lean 6σ phases are illustrated in figure 6-5.

Sigma is the standard deviation from the mean of measurements of defects in a normal distribution

$\sigma = \sqrt{\Sigma\,(x\text{-}x)^2 / n}$

$\sigma = 32\%$ defects

$2\sigma = 5\%$ defects

$3\sigma = 0.3\%$ defects

$4\sigma = 6$ defects per 100,000

$5\sigma = 6$ defects per 10m

$6\sigma = 2$ defects per billion

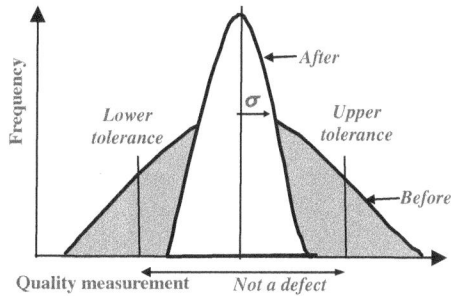

Figure 6-4: Sigma

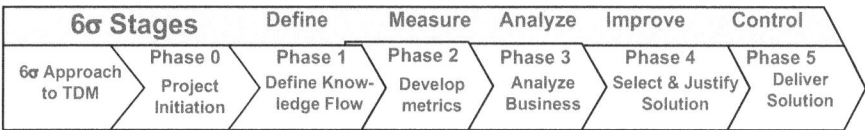

6σ Stages	Define	Measure	Analyze	Improve	Control
6σ Approach to TDM	Phase 0 Project Initiation	Phase 1 Define Knowledge Flow	Phase 2 Develop metrics	Phase 3 Analyze Business	Phase 4 Select & Justify Solution	Phase 5 Deliver Solution

Figure 6-5: Six Sigma Phases

Lean helps identify steps that don't add value and provides tools to eliminate them. It focuses on reducing waste and increasing process speed, Six Sigma improves the capability of steps that do add value. It focuses on reducing unwanted variation and improving the process capability of the value-added steps by spotlighting customer CTQs (critical to quality) as shown in Figure 6-6.

By enabling faster cycles of workflow and learning Lean Speed enables 6σ Quality. 6σ Quality enables Lean Speed because fewer defects means less time spent on rework.

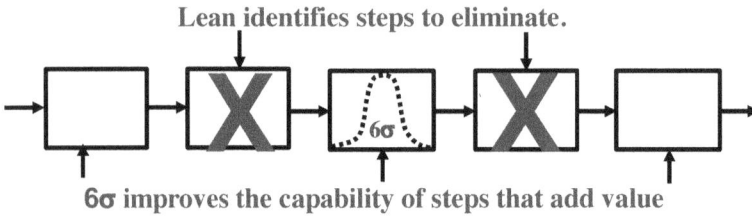

Lean identifies steps to eliminate.

6σ improves the capability of steps that add value

Figure 6-6: Lean Six Sigma

Value Proposition

Businesses depend on vast amounts of information that conventional IT systems often overlook - files, manuals, web pages, reports, letters and so on. We live in a world saturated with documents – but information alone does not guarantee success. It must be organized and catalogued for its intended purpose. Some of this information is embedded in document form on the web, on digital media, on paper or in employee skills and knowledge.

An enterprise must provide timely access to information and knowledge, distribute as need, re-use it when possible, realize opportunities and remove overhead. This means transforming the organization.

Process design and innovation coupled with technology to enhance work practice and looking at knowledge processing and flow to value across the entire firm provides insights into potential cost savings and efficiency gains. These include reduced costs, simpler and accelerated work processes, improved decision making, enhanced revenue and increased customer satisfaction. Consulting elements to achieve this are listed below.

Offer	Service Characteristics
Overview 0 EA (Executive Assessment)	A brief review and scoping of the major content-related issues and areas, and the business benefits from solving them. Does not go into detail apart from 'war stories'. Benefit: Helps the Client to justify further assessment of solutions; e.g., Content Strategy or Business Case
Axiom 1 DSP (Document Strategy & Policy Report)	Develops an overview of all content-related processes, systems and initiatives across the organization. Identifies major issues and potential solutions, estimates benefits and proposes a program of content, document and knowledge-related projects, including paper document management and archiving. Drafts the (content-related) strategic vision, identifies supporting policies, and identifies the processes and systems which need developing or changing to deliver this vision. Does not investigate costs, benefits, requirements or solutions in detail. Benefit: Helps the Client to justify and initiate a program to manage all content-related projects, with policies to implement the strategy
Axiom 2 SPI (Specification for Process Innovation)	Maps, analyses and benchmarks a business process together with the content flow supporting it. Inefficiencies are identified and their costs calculated. Proposals for process change are made together with the anticipated measurable benefits. The final deliverable is a master plan for business innovation that describes both the concept and its implementation. Benefit: Focuses on business process to identify improvements rather than fitting the process to the technology
Axiom 3 KWPA (Knowledge and Work Practice Assessment)	Creates a basis for managing knowledge flow, cultural practices and social capital. Produces a master action plan for business transformation of the way knowledge is shared and working practices managed. Benefit: Helps the Client to improve knowledge and work practices across process and system boundaries
Axiom 4 SRC (Solution Requirements Specification)	Defines business requirements for the user and the technical aspects of a service, linking processes to functions within an overall architecture. Benefit: Analyzes and specifies business requirements, before handing over to delivery for design, build and go live
Axiom 5 BC (Business Case)	Develops a detailed cost-benefit justification for a project, reviewing the current situation and identifying performance gaps. Specifies high level requirements and solutions if not already done. Benefit: Helps the Client to justify (or not) a specific project

Figure 6-7 shows the relationship of elements in the table while an overview of the consulting to establish a report is illustrated in Figure 6-8.

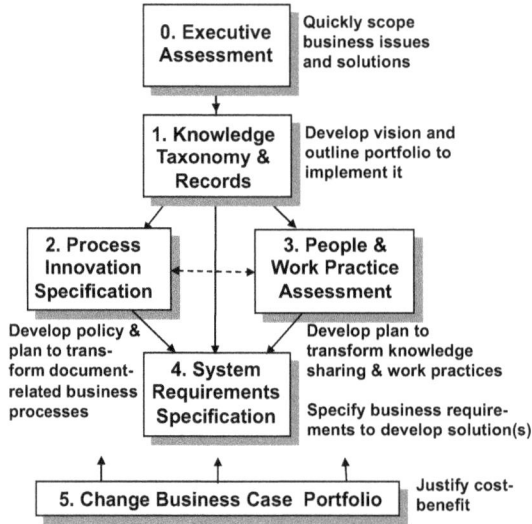

Figure 6-7: TDM report segments

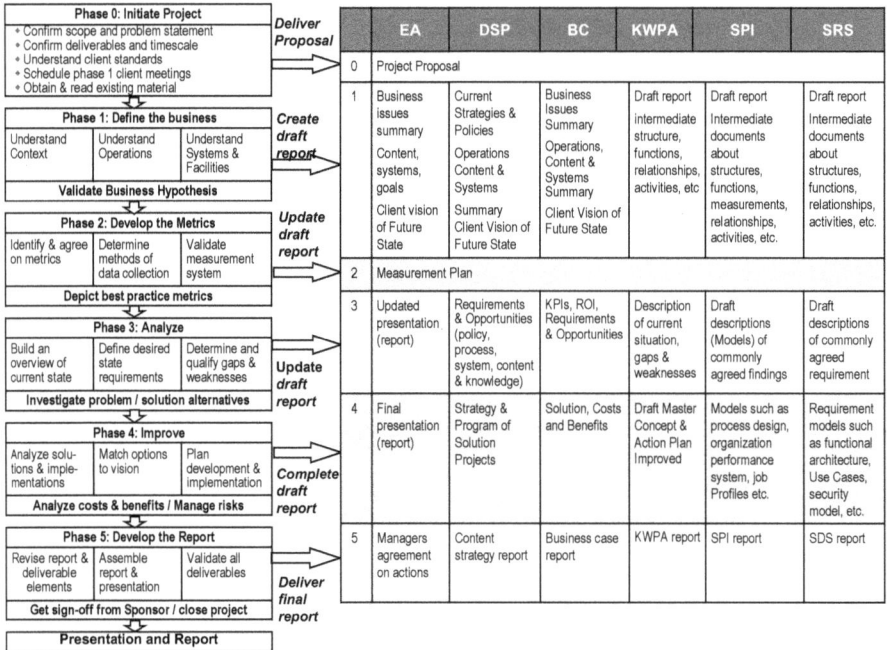

Figure 6-8: Developing the Report as a 6σ process

1. Executive Summary

2. Project Overview

2.1 Business Issues and Performance

2.2 Vision and Objectives

2.3 Preferred Solutions and
Recommendations

2.4 Implementation

2.5 Training Approach

2.6 Schedule

2.7 Costs and Benefits

2.8 Risks and Constraints

2.9 Project Team for next stage

2.10 Resources Required

2.11 Next Steps

3. Business Goals

3.1 Scorecard Performance Goals

  3.1.1 External Customers & Partners

  3.1.2 Internal Communities &
Operations

  3.1.3 Employees

  3.1.4 Financial and Market Share

3.2 Five Dimensions of Knowledge

4. Current State (not SRS)

4.1 Current Vision

4.2 Current Operations Summary

4.3 Current Processes and Content

4.4 Current Knowledge, Work
Practice and Culture

4.5 Current Technical Architecture
and Infrastructure

4.6 Current Change Initiatives

4.7 Expectations

4.8 Goals and Metrics

4.9 Analysis

5. Desired State

5.1 Desired State Vision and Policy

5.2 Desired State Process/Content

5.3 Desired State Knowledge, Work
Practice, Culture (CS, BC, KWPA)

5.4 Desired State Technical
Architecture

5.5 Solutions

5.6 Cost Benefit Analysis

5.7 Assumptions

5.8 Risk Management

6. Technology Requirements

6.1 System Overview (SRS)

6.2 System Components

6.3 Key Requirements

6.4 Quality Requirements

6.5 Integration with other systems

6.6 User Interface

6.7 Management and Support

6.8 Development and Implementation

6.9 Future development phases

7. Technical Requirements

7.1 Introduction – type of project

7.2 Knowledge Management

7.3 Records Management (EHR)

7.4 Workflow Management

8. Implementation Approach

8.1 Transition Principles

8.2 Schedule

  8.2.1 Phase 1: Key Activities

  8.2.2 Phase 2: Key Activities

  8.2.3 Phase 3: Key Activities

8.3 Program/ next stage project team

8.4 Resources required

8.5 Training Approach

8.6 Next steps

Glossary/Appendices/SOW

Problem: Healthcare poses a significant risk to national sustainability, with government and academic institutions highlighting it as a critical issue. A wellness framework offers a solution to address these challenges.

Purpose: To improve population health, quality of life, and efficiency in healthcare delivery by integrating social, medical, and technological resources into a comprehensive health system (review Chapter 2).

Objective: Ensure adequate resources and well-configured systems to enhance population health both in and out of hospitals.

Goal 8. Improve community health:

- **Target 5.1**: Ensure sufficient health system resources and staff to implement the transformation portfolio.
- **Target 5.2** Define and support regional social and medical entities.

Goal 9. Integrate in-hospital and out-of-hospital care in the region:

- **Target 5.3**: Ensure hospital systems meet regional medical requirements.
- **Target 5.4**: Reduce average time for in-patient flow-to-wellness time.

Program Scope

- **In Scope**: Implement a framework to improve population.
- **Out of Scope**: Limited to population health within the region.

Background

Figure 6-3 illustrated how knowledge is delivered to a hospital's value chain. Projects 5.4 and 5.5 are supported by the Care Model in Project 5.6.

Key Performance Indicators (KPIs)

1. **Funding Metrics:** Dollar value of grants and donations.
2. **Population Health:** Reduction in ER visits and improvement in wellness quotient.
3. **Operational Efficiency:** Time-to-diagnosis, cost reduction per citizen, and reduced admission rates.
4. **Research Impact:** Time-to-result for research outcomes and global impact of innovations.

Threats and Risks

- Insufficient funding and resources.
- Resistance to technological adoption and process changes.
- Delayed outcomes due to over-focus on planning and research.

Project 5.1 Market

Purpose: involve the organization in developing service requirements for the community not just in delivery services to "fix" ailments.

Objectives:

- Partner with physicians to identify services for quality hospital care and emergency service as well as home healthcare providers to ensure surrounding community members are better served.
- Educate the community in healthy habits and hospital services benefits.
- Define what the development team must produce and how much time they have to bring it to market.

Candidate Sub Projects

- Project 5.1.1 Understand patients, markets, and capabilities
- Project 5.1.2 Define community marketing strategy
- Project 5.1.3 Coordinate with social programs
- Project 5.1.4 Diagnose participants and plan care in Health Fairs
- Project 5.1.5 Solicit sources of revenue

Project 5.2 Develop

Purpose: assemble a program of projects that transitions the hospital from its current to a future state and researching drugs, techniques and tests.

Objectives:

- Do pure research into drug, equipment and procedures
- Configure, build and/or install medical equipment and technology.

Candidate Sub Projects

- Project 5.2.1 Configure portfolio
- Project 5.2.2 Set up Project Management Office
- Project 5.2.3 Oversee programs
- Project 5.2.4 Test market for new/revised services

Project 5.3 Purchase

Purpose: Purchase and deliver both medical and non-medical supplies from qualified suppliers.

Objective:

- Qualify and select suppliers by auditing their key processes and process management to ensure that they can deliver products and services.
- Negotiate, claims, and terms and conditions.

Candidate Sub Projects:

- Project 5.3.1 Define purchasing strategy
- Project 5.3.2 Qualify & select suppliers
- Project 5.3.3 Manage orders
- Project 5.3.4 Analyze usage
- Project 5.3.5 (Re)define quality processes

Project 5.4 Deliver (review Project 5.6)

Purpose: Deliver quality in-hospital patient care.

Objectives:

- Optimize patient flow to wellness.
- Make effective, efficient use of staff, resources, equipment and facilities.

Candidate Sub Projects

Project 5.4.1 Administer In-patient records & documents
Project 5.4.2 Diagnose In-patient & Plan Care
Project 5.4.3 Provide In-patient Intervention
Project 5.4.4 Provide In-patient Therapy
Project 5.4.5 Provide In-patient Custodial Care

Project 5.5 Maintain (review Project 5.6)

Purpose: Treat out-patients in the community with what appears to be very similar to in-patient treatment in "Deliver" where "Intervention" is much less intense in-hospital interventions (chemotherapy, dialysis and simple surgery, may be done in out-patient settings).

Objectives

- Disparate out-patient services share the same IT system
- Make effective use of telemedicine and a virtual emergency room.
- Coordinate a care team using telemedicine to provide diagnosis, custodial care and out-patient progress tracking.

Candidate Sub Projects

Project 5.5.1 Administer Out-patient records & documents
Project 5.5.2 Diagnose Out-patient & Plan Care
Project 5.5.3 Coordinate Out-patient Intervention
Project 5.5.4 Coordinate Out-patient Therapy
Project 5.5.5 Coordinate Out-patient Custodial Care
Project 5.5.6 Simulate and Optimize Patient Flow to Wellness

Purpose: Optimize a portfolio flow to wellness while making exceptional use of staff, equipment and facilities

Objective: Reduce unproductive patient wait times while improving quality of care

Background: How RFID Technology Improves Hospital Care

by K. S. Pasupathy and T. R. Hellmich Havard Business Publishing 31Dec2015

Mayo Clinic's Saint Mary's Hospital in Rochester, MN... illustrates the role that a simple technology (e.g., RFID system) and a multidiscipline team can play in improving quality and cost of care processes. The project was launched in 2013 and was fully integrated into emergency room operations at St. Mary's year-end 2015. The new infrastructure was a real-time-location (RTL) system with sensors and devices using RFID technology to track movement of and locate patients, staff, and equipment. High-density RFID readers were installed in the ceilings. All patients receive RFID wristbands when they register. Staff members have RFID chips in their badges. And equipment is tagged with RFID stickers. The ED-CELL team developed software to provide RFID data to staff.

The RTL system was integrated with existing information technology systems to provide a visual display of the locations of patients, key staff members, and equipment, and how long each has been at the current location. The location and duration information for all patients, staff members and equipment can also be obtained using an RTL system search tool. It to automates reporting to government agencies and regulatory bodies of key quality metrics and issues alerts when patients having waited too long for pain medication or without being seen.

Actions and Deliverables

- Culture: Provide training to make effective use of RFID technology.
- Content: Develop or purchase software to store operating statistics.
- Process: Input statistics into 6σ for continuous improvement.
- Architecture: RFID technology integral to all hospital operations.
- Infrastructure: Internet of Things is critical to effective RFID operations.
- Risk: Inadequate oversight monitoring simulation in real-time.

Work Breakdown Structure

- Attach RFID tags to every critical entity: equipment, staff, resources.
- Put fixed RFID readers in to scan every room in the hospital accurately.
- Tag every patient with an RFID tag.
- Define a process using a CDS to determine a path to patient wellness as defined in a project by a Value Stream Map (VSM).
- Develop software to locate patients by RFID tag to assess their position with respect to their Project VSM and to assess flow to wellness.
- Develop software to continuously assess a portfolio of patient projects to optimize patient flow and entity utilization.
- Use monitored data in Lean 6σ initiatives to optimize operations.

Metrics

- Average time of in-patient hospital stay.
- Percent patients released with intervention successfully complete.
- Percent of patients requiring readmittance.
- Quality of Care as rated in a 1-5 Likert scale by patients.
- Percent unproductive patient wait time.
- Percent patient projects withdrawn and reinserted into the portfolio.

Benefits

- Improved quality of care.
- Reduced patient waiting.
- Increased use of critical equipment.
- Reduced average in-patient stay.

The Care Model in Figure 6-10 provides a framework for defining the program of patient project and subsequent simulation.

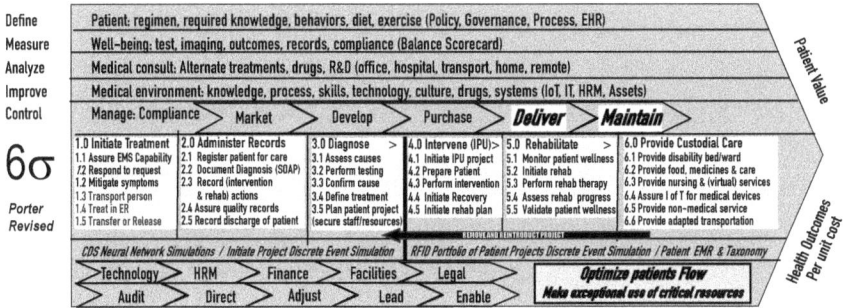

Figure 6-9: *Porter's Integrated Practice Unit Modified*

The lower-level activities listed in Table 6-3 are:

1.0 Initiate treatment	4.0 Intervene
1.1 Assure EMS capability	4.1 Initiate IPU project
1.2 Respond to request	4.2 Prepare patient
1.3 Mitigate symptoms	4.3 Perform intervention
1.4 Treat in ER	4.4 Initiate Recovery
1.5 Transfer or release	4.5 Initiate rehab plan
2.0 Administer records	5.0 Rehabilitate
2.1 Register patient for care	5.1 Monitor patient wellness
2.2 Document diagnosis (SOAP)	5.2 Initiate rehab
2.3 Record intervention & Rehab Act	5.3 Perform rehab therapy
2.4 Assure quality records	5.4 Assess rehab progress
2.5 Record discharge of patient	5.5 Validate patient wellness
3.0 Diagnose	6.0 Provide custodial care
3.1 Assess symptoms & anomalies	6.1 Provide disability bed/ward
3.2 Perform tests	6.2 Provide food, medications & personal care
3.3 Confirm cause	6.3 Provide nursing & (virtual) medical services
3.4 Define treatment	6.4 Provide IofT medical devices
3.5 Plan treatment	6.5 Provide adaptive transportation
(reserve staff/resources/facilities)	

Table 6-3: Healthcare Model Activities

- Michael Porter's IPU view (modified by the author) gives the impression that patients FLOW from one major activity to another.
- In fact, the majority of time spent by a patient is spent (bored and) waiting, some productive as in recovery and some unproductive as in waiting for a scarce resource (heart transplant), scarce staff (brain surgeon), scarce equipment (MRI machine) or scarce facility (OR).
- In some cases, all a patient does is wait while being monitored, fed and drugged (as for severe food poisoning).
- The most extensive activity in a patient project will usually be waiting.
- Therefore, value stream analysis where wait times are integral to the modeling process will be key to building a useful simulation.
- For medical facilities M. L. Dean calls this "Healing Pathway Analysis."
- How a patient is 'NURSED' while she or he 'WAIT' can have a significant impact on outcomes.
- For a simulation, the purpose is not to improve the quality of the process but to accurately predict the duration of equipment, resources, staff, and facilities required for patient intervention and wait to wellness.
- Analysis of the information derived from the simulation can subsequently be used to improve the quality and duration of the process using Value Stream Analysis (Another VSM) and Six Sigma.
- DRG (Diagnosis Related Group) is a Medicare payment classification system that groups clinically similar conditions that require similar amounts of inpatient resources.
- Medicare pays a pre-defined amount for all healthcare costs based on the hospital assigned DRG to a stay.
- This DRG includes payment for all services received while in the hospital (e.g., x-rays, MRIs and any surgeries). It also includes any supplies you use (e.g., bandages, alcohol swabs or bedpans).
- Hospitals don't bill for every item or service it provides, because it's all rolled up into the DRG based payment.

Figure 6-10 from The Institute for Healthcare Improvement (modified by the author) provides a view of flow between critical and waiting events. The hospital is divided into Critical Intervention zones and 6 WAIT zones.

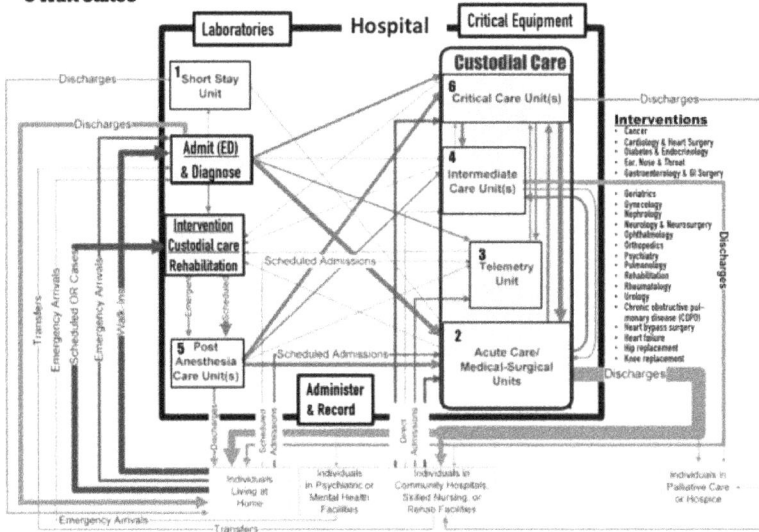

Figure 6-10: Patient Wait States

Patient Value Stream Map

Patient Project is a value stream as shown in Figure 6-11 of waiting and passing through event zones. Given that event zones will have average and variation times based on their use, the objective is to compute the wait times between event zones where the patient is competing for access to scarce resource, equipment and facility associated with the events with other patients. Based on the intervention, a patient will have a priority of 1-3 assigned for access to an event zone.

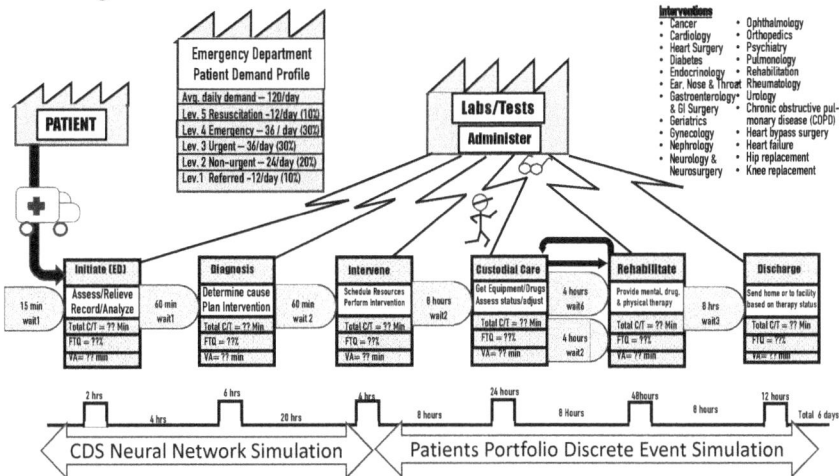

Figure 6-11: Patient Value Stream Map

MCC = Major Complications or Comorbidities

DRG 470: Major Joint Replacement Without MCC:

- Initiate: Pre-op assessments, patient admitted.
- Diagnosis: Confirmation of need for joint replacement.
- Intervene: Anesthesia consultation, surgical team preparation; joint replacement surgery.
- Custodial care: Initial recovery in PACU (Post-Anesthesia Care Unit).
- Rehabilitate: Early mobilization, physical Rehabilitation.
- Discharge: Patient discharge, ambulating independently, pain managed.
- Post Discharge: Rehabilitation, check-ups.

DRG 871: Septicemia or Severe Sepsis Without Mechanical Ventilation:

- Initiate: Emergency or inpatient admission with suspected sepsis.
- Diagnosis: Blood tests, cultures, vital sign monitoring.
- Intervene: Broad-spectrum antibiotics, fluid resuscitation.
- Custodial care: Frequent vital sign checks, lab test to monitor response.
- Rehab: Adjust antibiotics based on culture results to manage symptoms.
- Discharge: On antibiotics, stabilized, vital signs and no infection.
- Post Discharge: Outpatient lab work to ensure infection resolution.

DRG 91: Heart Failure and Shock with MCC:

- Initiate: ER or direct admission due to heart failure.
- Diagnosis: Echocardiogram, lab tests, chest X-ray.
- Intervene: Diuretics, oxygen therapy, medication adjustments.
- Custodial care: Vital signs, fluid balance, kidney function.
- Rehabilitate: Condition stabilization; patient responding to treatment.
- Discharge: Patient educated on diet, medications, retaining fluids.
- Post Discharge: home monitoring.

DRG 194: Simple Pneumonia with MCC:

- Initiate: ER or inpatient admission due to suspected pneumonia.
- Diagnosis: Chest X-ray, blood tests, sputum cultures.
- Intervene: Antibiotic therapy (IV or oral).
- Custodial care: Vital signs, oxygen levels, response to antibiotics.
- Rehabilitate: Improvement in respiratory status, resolution of fever.
- Discharge: When stable, tolerating and education on antibiotics.
- Post Discharge: Outpatient check-up for recovery confirmation.

DRG 065: Intracranial Hemorrhage or Cerebral Infarction with MCC:

- Initiate: ER or urgent inpatient admission due to stroke.
- Diagnosis: CT scan, MRI to assess bleeding or infarct.
- Intervene: Stabilization, BP control, possible surgical intervention.
- Custodial care: Neurological checks, ICU monitoring if necessary.
- Rehabilitate: Stabilized, stroke symptoms managed, physical, occupational, speech therapy.
- Discharge: Based on recovery. medical stability, rehab, home care plan.
- Post-discharge follow-up: Neurological follow-up, outpatient rehab.

DRG 871: Septicemia or Severe Sepsis Without Mechanical Ventilation:

- Initiate: ER or inpatient transfer: triage, blood culture, vital signs check.
- Diagnosis: Blood work, cultures, lactate levels, imaging if necessary.
- Intervene: broad-spectrum IV antibiotics and fluids immediately.
- Custodial care: Continuous (vital signs, urine output, BP); adjust fluids.
- Rehabilitate: adjust antibiotics; remove source of infection.
- Discharge: Home or outpatient facility when clinically stable and infection controlled.
- Post-Discharge: Follow-up with GP or infectious disease specialist.

DRG 189: Pulmonary Edema and Respiratory Failure:

- Initiate: ER, admission: vital signs, oxygen levels, arterial blood gas.
- Diagnosis: Chest X-ray, echocardiogram, lab tests.
- Intervene: Oxygen therapy, diuretics, ventilation if needed.
- Custodial care: Continuous pulse oximetry, fluid output, blood gases.
- Rehabilitate: Improvement in respiratory function; off ventilation.
- Discharge Planning: Respiration stabilizes; home or rehab for recovery.
- Post-Discharge: Outpatient follow-up for respiratory function.

DRG 683: Renal Failure with MCC:

- Initiate: ER or direct nephrology referral: blood work, urine.
- Diagnosis: GFR, creatinine clearance, imaging; acute vs. chronic.
- Intervene: Manage IV fluids, electrolyte dialysis.
- Custodial care: Fluid out, vital signs: frequent lab tests, adjust fluids, diuretics, or dialysis.
- Stabilization: Stable creatinine, electrolyte levels, and not dialysis.
- Discharge: Once kidney function stabilizes or home or outpatient dialysis schedule set.
- Post-Discharge: Nephrology follow-up to monitor kidney function.

DRG 25: Percutaneous Cardiovascular Procedures Without MCC:

- Initiate: Scheduled or ER; pre-op labs, EKG, cardiac risk assessment.
- Diagnosis: Angiography, EKG, stress test result; confirm stent need.
- Intervene: Angioplasty, stent placement; perform procedure.
- Custodial care: Post-op EKG, monitoring for complications; adjust meds/anticoagulants.
- Rehabilitate: Stable cardiac function, no recurrent symptoms.
- Discharge: If stable, on proper medications; home with medication plan.
- Post-Discharge: Cardiology follow-up for EKG, stress test, stent success, no complications.

DRG 193: Simple Pneumonia Without MCC:

- Initiate: ER or direct admission; chest X-ray, blood tests.
- Diagnosis: Confirm pneumonia via X-ray, sputum culture; Initiate antibiotics.
- Intervene: IV antibiotics, fluids, oxygen; administer antibiotics based on culture.
- Custodial care: Decrease in fever, improvement in lung function; oral antibiotics.
- Rehabilitate: Once stable and fever-free.
- Discharge: education on completing antibiotics; home with follow-up for chest X-ray.
- Post-Discharge: Outpatient follow-up to ensure infection resolution.

DRG 853: Infectious & Parasitic Diseases with O.R. Procedure with MCC:

- Initiate: Emergency Room; lab tests, cultures, imaging; infection severity.
- Diagnosis: Confirm infection source (e.g., abscess, osteomyelitis); prepare for surgery.
- Intervene: Surgery to remove infection source; perform operation.
- Custodial care: Post-op recovery, wound care; adjust antibiotics, manage wound healing.
- Rehabilitate: Improvement in infection markers, wound healing; oral antibiotics.
- Discharge: Wound healing complete or manageable; educate; home or long-term care.
- Post-Discharge: Follow-up to ensure infection resolution.

DRG 280: Acute Myocardial Infarction, Discharged Alive with MCC:

- Initiate: ER with chest pain; EKG, cardiac enzymes.
- Diagnosis: Confirm heart attack with troponin levels, EKG; initiate treatment.
- Intervene: Percutaneous coronary intervention (PCI) or thrombolytics.
- Custodial care: continuous EKG, blood pressure, and heart function; manage risk.
- Rehabilitate: Improved cardiac function; (anticoagulants, beta-blockers).
- Discharge: Stable heart function; medication education, cardiac rehab schedule.
- Post-Discharge: Scheduled cardiologist follow-up for EKG, stress test.

DRG 286: Circulatory Disorders with Cardiac Catheterization with MCC:

- Initiate: ER or scheduled admission; pre-op tests (labs, EKG).
- Diagnosis: Catheterization lab imaging (angiogram); confirm vascular blockage.
- Intervene: Cardiac catheterization (with or without stent); perform the procedure.
- Custodial care: Post-procedure EKG, vital signs, catheter site checks.
- Rehabilitate: Stable cardiac function; transition to medical therapy.
- Discharge: Stable heart function, no complications; educate, home.
- Post-Discharge: Cardiologist follow-up with stress tests and imaging.

DRG 327: Stomach, Esophageal, and Duodenal Procedures with MCC:

- Initiate: Scheduled or ER due to upper GI issues (bleeding, obstruction, cancer, ulcers).
- Diagnosis: Endoscopy, biopsy, or imaging (CT, X-ray); yes/no to surgical intervention.
- Intervene: Consultation, anesthesia., secure consent, NPO, IV fluids; Surgical team performs stomach, esophageal, or duodenal procedure.
- Custodial care (PACU): Recovery room, initial monitoring; ICU or Med-Surg.
- Rehabilitate: Physical therapy, post-surgery diet (liquid to soft food).
- Discharge: Patient diet stabilized, pain managed, complication free, home or rehab facility.
- Post-discharge: Gastroenterology or surgical follow-up 2 weeks.

DRG 177: Respiratory Infections & Inflammations with MCC:

- Initiate: ER or direct admission due to severe respiratory symptoms.
- Diagnosis: Lab results, imaging, X-ray, clinical exam.
- Intervene: Start IV antibiotics or antivirals, oxygen ventilation, fluids.
- Custodial care: Vital signs, ABGs, oxygen saturation, urine output; adjust oxygen antibiotic
- Rehabilitate: Improvement in symptoms, lung function, vital signs.
- Discharge: Clinical stabilization, improved oxygen requirements, infection controlled, home with oral antibiotics or transfer to rehab.
- Post-discharge Follow-up: Outpatient pulmonary or infectious disease specialist follow-up.
- Patient Flow: Emergency Department or Direct Admission → Radiology/Imaging → ICU/Step-down → Operating Room → PACU → Med/Surg Unit → Rehab → Case Management → Discharge.

Critical Hospital Entities

In a hospital, critical job classes, equipment, facilities, laboratories, and therapies/interventions are essential for comprehensive patient care:

1. Critical Job Classes

- Physicians & Surgeons: GPs, & Specialists (cardiology, oncology, neurology, surgery, etc.
- Nurses: Provide patient care, administer medication, and monitor patient health.
- Anesthesiologists: Manage anesthesia during surgeries and other procedures.
- Radiologists: Interpret medical images and assist in diagnosing conditions.
- Pharmacists: Dispense medications and advise on their use.
- Medical Technologists/Laboratory Technicians: Conduct laboratory tests and analyses.
- Physical Therapists: Assist patients in recovering mobility and function.
- Occupational Therapists: Help patients regain skills needed for daily living.
- Respiratory Therapists: Provide care for patients with breathing difficulties.
- EMTs & Paramedics: Provide emergency care and transport.
- Hospital Admin: Manage hospital operations and ensure compliance with regulations.
- Support Staff: Includes housekeeping, food services, and maintenance personnel who ensure the hospital's smooth functioning.

2. Critical Equipment

- MRI and CT Scanners: Used for detailed imaging of the body.
- X-ray Machines: Provide imaging for diagnosing fractures, infections, and other conditions.
- Ultrasound Machines: Used for imaging soft tissues, blood flow, and during pregnancy.
- ECG/EKG Machines: Monitor heart activity.
- Ventilators: Provide respiratory support to patients.
- Defibrillators: Used to restore normal heart rhythm in emergencies.
- Surgical Instruments: Essential tools for performing surgeries.
- Infusion Pumps: Administer medications, fluids, and nutrients.
- Dialysis Machines: Provide renal support for patients with kidney failure.
- Patient Monitors: Vital signs such as heart rate, blood pressure, oxygen saturation.
- Heart by-pass machine.
- Dialysis Machine.

3. Critical Facilities

- Emergency Room (ER): Provides immediate care for acute injuries and illnesses.
- Intensive Care Unit (ICU): Offers specialized care for critically ill patients.
- Operating Rooms (ORs): Equipped for surgical procedures.
- Labor and Delivery Rooms: For childbirth and related care.
- Radiology Department: Houses imaging equipment like MRI, CT, and X-rays.
- Pharmacy: Dispenses medications and advises on their use.
- Laboratories: Diagnostic tests, including blood work, microbiology, and pathology.

4. Ubiquitous Facilities

- Inpatient Wards: Accommodate patients requiring overnight stays.
- Outpatient Clinics: Provide routine care and follow-up appointments.

5. Critical Laboratories

- Chemistry Laboratory: Analyzes blood and other body fluids for chemical components.
- Hematology Laboratory: Studies blood and its disorders.
- Microbiology Laboratory: Identifies infectious organisms and conducts antimicrobial susceptibility testing.
- Pathology Laboratory: Examines tissue samples for disease diagnosis.
- Blood Bank: Collects, stores, and supplies blood and blood products.
- Immunology Laboratory: Tests for immune disorders and allergies.
- Molecular Diagnostics Laboratory: Conducts genetic testing and molecular diagnostics.

6. Critical Therapies and Interventions

- Surgical Interventions.
- General Surgery: Broad range of surgeries including appendectomy, gallbladder removal, and hernia repairs.
- Cardiothoracic Surgery: Involves heart and lung surgeries, such as coronary artery bypass grafting (CABG).
- Neurosurgery: Focuses on surgeries of the brain and spinal cord.
- Orthopedic Surgery: Involves the musculoskeletal system, including joint replacements and fracture repairs.
- Plastic and Reconstructive Surgery: Cosmetic and restorative surgeries.
- Transplant Surgery: Transplanting organs like kidneys, liver, or heart.

7. Pharmaceutical Interventions

- Antibiotics: For treating bacterial infections.
- Chemotherapy: For treating cancer.
- Antivirals: For treating viral infections.
- Analgesics: For pain management.
- Anticoagulants: For preventing blood clots.
- Vaccinations: For preventing diseases.
- Immunotherapy: For treating certain cancers and autoimmune diseases.

8. Other Therapies

- Radiation Therapy: Uses high-energy radiation to treat cancer.
- Physical Therapy: Rehab for injury recovery and improving function.
- Occupational Therapy: Helps patients regain independence in activities.
- Speech Therapy: Assists patients with speech and swallowing disorders.
- Respiratory Therapy: Provides care for patients with breathing issues.
- Nutritional Therapy: Manages diet and nutrition.
- **Other Critical Areas**: Sterilization Unit; Intensive Care for Neonates (NICU); Burn Unit: Rehabilitation Center.

Given that the journey of an ill patient through a hospital from initiation to recovery involves a well-coordinated flow through various interventions and therapies depending on the patient's condition:

1. Admission and Initial Assessment

- Emergency Room (ER) or Outpatient Clinic: The patient typically arrives at the ER for acute or urgent issues or for non-emergent concerns. Triage is conducted to prioritize care based on the severity.
- Initial Assessment: A Practitioner performs a preliminary assessment, including vital signs, medical history, and symptoms.
- Diagnostic Tests: Initial tests such as blood work, imaging (X-rays, CT scans, MRI), and other diagnostics may be ordered to determine the underlying condition.

2. Diagnosis and Care Planning

- Consultation with Specialists: Based on initial findings, the patient may be referred to specialists (e.g., cardiologist, neurologist, surgeon) for a more detailed evaluation.
- Diagnosis: After analyzing the test results and assessments, a diagnosis is made. This may involve further diagnostic procedures such as biopsies, endoscopies, or advanced imaging.
- Care Plan Development: A personalized treatment plan is developed, which could include surgical interventions, pharmaceutical therapies, or other therapeutic measures. The care team, including doctors, nurses, and specialists, collaborates to design this plan.

3. Interventions and Therapies

Medical Management

- Pharmaceutical Therapy: Medications are prescribed to manage symptoms, treat infections, or address underlying conditions. This might include antibiotics, antivirals, pain management drugs, or chronic disease management medications (e.g., insulin for diabetes).
- Monitoring and Support: Continuous monitoring (e.g., heart rate, blood pressure, oxygen saturation) is done in wards or specialized units like the ICU if needed. Supportive care, including IV fluids, oxygen therapy, and nutritional support, is provided.

Surgical Interventions

- Pre-Operative Care: If surgery is required, the patient undergoes pre-operative preparations, including anesthesia evaluation, fasting, and consent procedures.
- Surgery: The surgery is performed in an operating room by a specialized surgical team.
- Post-Operative Care: After surgery, the patient is transferred to a recovery room or ICU for close monitoring. Pain management, wound care, and prevention of complications are prioritized.

Therapies and Rehabilitation

- Physical Therapy: Initiated to help the patient regain mobility and strength, especially after surgery or prolonged illness.
- Occupational Therapy: Focuses on helping the patient regain independence in daily activities.
- Respiratory Therapy: For patients with respiratory issues, breathing exercises, and ventilatory support might be provided.
- Nutritional Therapy: A dietitian may be involved to ensure the patient receives proper nutrition tailored to their condition.

4. Monitoring and Adjustment (Custodial Care)

- Regular Assessments: The patient's progress is regularly monitored through clinical evaluations, repeat imaging, or lab tests. This helps in assessing the effectiveness of the treatment plan.
- Adjustments to Treatment: Based on the patient's response, medications might be adjusted, additional therapies introduced, or changes in the care plan implemented.

5. Discharge Planning

- Discharge Evaluation: Once the patient is stable and showing signs of recovery, the care team assesses readiness for discharge. This includes ensuring the patient can manage at home or needs rehabilitation.
- Education and Instructions: The patient and their family receive instructions on medication, follow-up appointments, and lifestyle modifications. This might also include wound care, physical therapy exercises, or dietary restrictions.
- Follow-Up Care: Arrangements are made for follow-up appointments, either with their GP, specialists, or outpatient rehab facilities.

6. Post-Discharge and Long-Term Recovery

- Home Care: Some patients may require home health services, such as nursing care, physical therapy, or assistance with daily activities.
- Outpatient Rehabilitation: For patients needing continued physical, occupational, or speech therapy, outpatient services are provided.
- Long-Term Management: Chronic conditions may require ongoing management through regular visits to specialists, lifestyle modifications, and adherence to prescribed medications.

7. Return to Wellness

- Final Assessments: As patients continue to recover, they undergo final assessments to ensure they have regained sufficient function & health.
- Full Recovery or Management of Chronic Conditions: Ideally, the patient returns to their previous state of health or adjusts to a new baseline of wellness with manageable chronic conditions.
- Ongoing Support: Continued support may be needed, such as counseling, support groups, or regular check-ups to prevent relapse or manage long-term effects of their condition.

Context: a patient stay in hospital is represented as a project by a Lean Value Stream Map and the hospital is represented by:

- 6 ubiquitous wait care zones (1. Short Term, 2. Medical-Surgical, 3. Telemetry, 4, Interim, 5. Post Operation, 6. Intensive Care), and
- Scarce zones like MRI, X-ray, surgical, chemotherapy, dialysis, diagnostic, lab, and rehab facilities, and
- a resource can vary from a titanium hip to a new heart, and equipment can vary from a surgical tool kit to heart by-pass machine.

Question: how can a portfolio of all the patient projects be modelled as Lean Value Streams based on Medicare DRGs flowing through the hospital zones considering that each patient has varying degrees of priority (e.g. heart attack, benign tumor removal, etc.) to predict a timeline for each patient and nurse, physician, non-medical staff, resource, equipment and zone requirements for each 24-hour day for the next five days?

To model a portfolio of patient projects as Lean Value Streams, flowing through hospital zones while considering varying patient priorities and resource constraints, each patient is represented as a "project" with specific resource and zone requirements. We can use Python to create a simulation model, where each patient passes through different hospital zones over time. Critical resources like medical staff, equipment, and zones are constrained, meaning that delays might occur if resources are unavailable.

Steps to Model the Portfolio of Patient Projects:

1. Define Zones: Represent the hospital zones (ER, ICU, Operating Rooms, etc.) as stages in the Value Stream. Some zones are ubiquitous (always available), while others are scarce (limited).

2. Define Resources: Resources include nurses, physicians, equipment, and specialized staff, each with limited availability. Some equipment may be shared across multiple patients (e.g., MRI machines)

3. Define Priorities: Prioritize patients based on severity of condition (e.g., heart attacks have higher priority than benign tumor removal).

4. Track Time: Estimate the time spent by each patient in each zone based on their condition and resource availability.

5. Predict Resource Requirements: For each day over the next five days, predict the resource usage based on the number of patients in hospital.

Key Concepts in the Program:

1. Patient Flow: Patients are transitioned through hospital zones based on their priority and resource availability.

2. Resource Management: For each patient, resources like nurses and physicians are checked for availability. If sufficient resources are available, the patient transitions to the next zone.

3. Simulation: The process is simulated for a number of days (5 days in this case), predicting the resource usage for each day.

4. Output: The simulation results are stored in a DataFrame, showing the final state of each patient.

Sample Python Simulation Programs

```python
python
import numpy as np
import pandas as pd
import random
# Constants
NUM_DAYS = 5
NUM_PATIENTS = 100  # Simulate 100 patients
TIME_PERIODS = NUM_DAYS * 24  # 24 hours each day
ZONES = ['ER', 'Medical-Surgical', 'Telemetry', 'Interim', 'Post Operation', 'ICU', 'MRI', 'X-ray', 'Surgery', 'Rehab']
RESOURCE_TYPES = ['Nurse', 'Physician', 'Surgeon', 'Technician', 'Equipment']
# Create patient priorities (higher value = more urgent)
priorities = ['low', 'medium', 'high']
patient_data = pd.DataFrame({
    'patient_id': range(1, NUM_PATIENTS + 1),
    'priority': np.random.choice(priorities, NUM_PATIENTS, p=[0.4, 0.4, 0.2]),
    'current_zone': np.random.choice(ZONES, NUM_PATIENTS),
    'time_spent': np.random.randint(1, 4, NUM_PATIENTS)  # Hours already spent in zone
})
# Resource availability (randomly set availability for each resource type)
resource_availability = {
    'Nurse': random.randint(10, 20),
    'Physician': random.randint(5, 10),
    'Surgeon': random.randint(3, 5),
    'Technician': random.randint(10, 15),
    'Equipment': random.randint(10, 20)  # General purpose equipment
}
# Define function to calculate patient zone transitions based on priority
```

```python
def transition_patient(patient, resource_availability):
    current_zone = patient['current_zone']
    priority = patient['priority']
    # Determine next zone based on current zone and priority
    if current_zone == 'ER':
        next_zone = 'ICU' if priority == 'high' else 'Medical-Surgical'
    elif current_zone == 'Medical-Surgical':
        next_zone = 'Telemetry' if priority == 'medium' else 'Interim'
    elif current_zone == 'Surgery':
        next_zone = 'Post Operation'
    else:
        next_zone = 'Rehab' if priority == 'low' else 'Discharge'
    # Check resource availability in the next zone
    if resource_availability['Nurse'] > 0 and resource_availability['Physician'] > 0:
        # Reduce available resources
        resource_availability['Nurse'] -= 1
        resource_availability['Physician'] -= 1
        return next_zone
    else:
        return current_zone  # Stay in current zone if resources are unavailable
# Simulate patient flow through hospital over time
def simulate_patient_flow(patient_data, resource_availability, num_days):
    for day in range(num_days):
        for patient_id, patient in patient_data.iterrows():
            # Transition patients based on priority and resource availability
            patient_data.loc[patient_id, 'current_zone'] = transition_patient(patient,
resource_availability)
            patient_data.loc[patient_id, 'time_spent'] += 1
# Increment time spent in the current zone
        # Print daily resource usage summary
        print(f"Day {day + 1} Resource Usage: {resource_availability}")
    return patient_data
# Run the simulation for the specified number of days
final_patient_data    =    simulate_patient_flow(patient_data,    resource_availability,
NUM_DAYS)
# Display the final state of patients
print(final_patient_data)
# Save the final data to a CSV file
final_patient_data.to_csv('patient_flow_simulation.csv', index=False)
```

This approach can be expanded to include more detailed model of equipment, staff schedules, more zones, and stochastic events like emergencies or equipment failures.

Multiple simulations are required to simulate patient flow and entity utilization in a hospital.

- Given age, gender, comorbidity level, symptoms, mitigate the symptoms and propose a cause.
- Determine the cause, propose alternative intervention plans using a Neural Network Simulation.
- Given alternative interventions, determine the appropriate intervention, with a severity level and an intervention project plan as a Value Stream Map with past average, minimum and maximum durations of critical entity usage.
- Introduce the project into a real-time portfolio of current patient projects to schedule and determine availability of critical staff, resources, equipment and facilities, to calculate wait times between critical events and update Patient Project estimates using DES.
- Using an RFID wrist band to track the transition of the patient through the project plan.
- Introduce the patient project into the portfolio where all patients are tracked with RFIDs to continuously update actual use of critical areas and times in queues using DES to optimize patient flow and reschedule critical entities if necessary to optimize their use.
- In addition to transitioning patients to wellness, use data gathered from continuously simulated operations as input to a Lean Six Sigma Methodology to optimize hospital delivery services.

After the first diagnosis, a repair may be simple, 'set a broken bone' or not, 'open heart surgery.' Two thirds of the hospital's patients are out-patient with no overnight stay. In-patient stay median is 5 days, minimum of 1 day and maximum of months (heart transplant).

To create a comprehensive simulation of hospital patient flow and resource utilization to meet each requirement, each component and its role is explained with an outline of the corresponding Python code.

Step-by-Step Simulation Objectives and Components

1. Patient Diagnosis and Treatment Proposal: For each patient, given age, gender, comorbidities, and symptoms, simulate symptom mitigation and propose a probable cause using a neural network simulation (NNS).

2. Alternative Treatment Plans: Based on the diagnosis, use NNS to propose alternative interventions.

3. Intervention Project Planning: Use Value Stream Mapping (VSM) to define critical stages, estimate resource utilization, and assign a severity level and expected duration.

4. Real-Time Scheduling: Integrate each patient project with current resource utilization in the hospital. Update the plan based on resource availability and critical event wait times using DES.

5. Patient Flow Tracking: Use RFIDs and adjust schedules in real-time.

6. Lean Six Sigma Optimization: Use gathered data to improve hospital workflows and reduce wait times.

Step 1: Patient Diagnosis and Initial Symptom Mitigation using a Neural Network Model, to predict a probable cause based on inputs like age, gender, comorbidity level, and symptoms. Here is a simplified NNS to predict a probable cause:

```python
python
import tensorflow as tf
from tensorflow.keras import layers, models
import numpy as np
# Sample patient data - age, gender (0=female, 1=male), comorbidity level, symptoms
X = np.array([[35, 1, 2, 3], [50, 0, 3, 5], [65, 1, 1, 4], [30, 0, 0, 2]])  # Example input data
y = np.array([0, 1, 0, 1])  # Example labels (0=simple case, 1=complex case)
# Define Neural Network model
model = models.Sequential([
    layers.Dense(10, activation='relu', input_shape=(4,)),
    layers.Dense(10, activation='relu'),
    layers.Dense(2, activation='softmax')  # Two output classes for simplicity
])
model.compile(optimizer='adam', loss='sparse_categorical_crossentropy', metrics=['accuracy'])
model.fit(X, y, epochs=10)
# Predicting for a new patient
new_patient = np.array([[40, 1, 2, 4]])
probable_cause = np.argmax(model.predict(new_patient))
print("Predicted probable cause:", probable_cause)
```

Step 2: Generate Alternative Intervention Plans using the initial diagnosis enhanced and NNS to recommend treatment pathways.

```python
python
# Define alternative intervention plans for a patient based on probable cause
def suggest_interventions(cause):
    if cause == 0:
        return ["Splinting", "Physical Therapy"]
    elif cause == 1:
        return ["Cardiac Monitoring", "Surgery", "Rehabilitation"]
    else:
        return ["Consult Specialist"]
interventions = suggest_interventions(probable_cause)
print("Suggested Interventions:", interventions)
```

Step 3: Define an Intervention with a Value Stream Map (VSM) Project Plan using simpy to simulate the patient's treatment path as a series of events based on the intervention plan to estimated time and entity usage of each step in the VSM.

```python
python
import simpy
# Environment setup
env = simpy.Environment()
# Define resources
doctors = simpy.Resource(env, capacity=5)
nurses = simpy.Resource(env, capacity=10)
# Define patient intervention project plan based on VSM
def intervention_project(env, name, interventions, doctors, nurses):
    for intervention in interventions:
        with doctors.request() as request:
            yield request
            duration = np.random.normal(30, 5)  # Assume interventions take ~30 min
            print(f"{name} starts {intervention} at {env.now:.2f}")
            yield env.timeout(duration)
            print(f"{name} completes {intervention} at {env.now:.2f}")
# Start simulation
patient_intervention = env.process(intervention_project(env, "Patient 1", interventions, doctors, nurses))
env.run()
```

Step 4: Real-Time Scheduling with DES for Resource Allocation: Each patient's project is integrated into the hospital portfolio, scheduling resources based on availability and adjusting times for critical events.

python
```
def patient_generator(env, doctors, nurses):
    i = 0
    while True:
        yield env.timeout(np.random.exponential(10))  # New patient every ~10 minutes
        i += 1
        interventions = suggest_interventions(np.random.randint(0, 2))
        env.process(intervention_project(env, f"Patient {i}", interventions, doctors, nurses))
# Run the environment with continuous patient arrivals
env.process(patient_generator(env, doctors, nurses))
env.run(until=480)  # Run for an 8-hour shift
```

Step 5: Patient Tracking Using an RFID track each patient's location and resource usage, dynamically updating schedules based on their progress through the intervention project. This tracking can be represented in the simulation by updating the patient's progress and recalculating resource availability in simpy.

Step 6: Continuous Data Collection for Lean Six Sigma Optimization
Simulated data from each patient's flow is collected to evaluate and optimize throughput, minimize waste, and reduce wait times.
Lean Six Sigma process uses metrics like:
1] Average wait time per stage;
2] Resource utilization rates;
3] number of interventions successfully completed within estimated time.

This simulation structure offers a realistic approach to dynamically manage and optimize hospital workflows, continuously adapting to each patient need and responding to real-time demand and resource availability.

Note: this is an ongoing project; more work needs to be done to clarify and refine the simulations. Also, this precedes work necessary to integrate it into HIT and ERP systems. Both the neural network and discrete event simulations will require a great deal of data within those systems.

BIBLIOGRAPHY

- Audi, Robert, *Epistemology*, Routledge, 1998.
- Amadeo, Kimberly Amadeo, *The rising cost of health care by year and its causes*, https://www.thebalance.com/causes-of-rising-healthcare-costs-4064878, 2018.
- American Productivity & Quality Centre, Process Classification Framework.
- Beer, Stafford, *The Heart of Enterprise*, John Wiley & Sons Ltd, 1979.
- Bowron C., MD and Cummings, M., MD, *How doctors should think: Heuristic thinking isn't heretical*, www.kevinmd.com/blog, Feb 2018.
- Carnegie Mellon SEI, People Capability Maturity Model.
- Davenport, T.H., *Process Innovation*, HBS Press, 1993.
- Deming, W. Edwards, *The New Economics*. M.I.T. Press. 2000.
- Drucker, Peter F., *Managing for the Future*, Truman Talley Books/Dutton, 1992.
- Goldratt, E., *The Goal*, Creative Output, 1984.
- Hammer, Michael, Champy, James, *Reengineering the Corporation*, Harper Collins, 1993.
- Harris, A. and Sharma, A., *The Future of Health and Aged Care Expenditure In Australia* by Centre For Health Economics Draft, Monash University, Working Paper No 2016-05, 16 June 2016.
- Hopp, W.J., and Spearman, M.L., *Factory Physics*, Irwin, 1996.
- International Standard Organization, *ISO 15489 Records Management Standard*.
- Jones, Jeffrey I., *Collective Social Intelligence*, 2017, Austin Macauley Publisher, Ltd. London.
- Jones, Jim I., *Document Methodology*, 1999, II 2007, III 2020.
- Kaplan, R. and Norton, D., *Using the Balanced Scorecard as a Strategic Management System*, Harvard Business Review, Jul-Aug 2007.
- Kuhn, Thomas S., *The Structure of Scientific Revolutions*, University of Chicago Press, 1962.
- Lynn, Joanne, MD, *Medicaring Communities,* Createspace, June 2016.
- Makary, Marty, *The Price We Pay*, Bloomsbury Publishing, 2019

- Porter, Michael E. and Teisberg, Elizabeth O., *Redefining Healthcare*, HBS Press, 2006.
- Porter, Michael E., *Competitive Advantage*, The Free Press, Macmillan, 1985.
- Pritsker, A. A. B. Sigal, C.E., and Hammesfahr, R.D., *SLAM II Network Models for Decision Support*, Prentice-Hall, 1989.
- Project Management Institute, Portfolio, Program and Project Standards, 2013.
- Pyzdek, Thomas, *The Six Sigma Handbook Version IV*, McGraw Hill, 2014.
- Reid, T. R., *The Healing of America*, The Penguin Press, 2009.
- Richards, Chet, *Certain to Win John Boyd's Strategy in the 21st Century*, J. Addams & Partners, Inc., March 2005.
- Ross, Douglas, An Introduction to SADT Structured Analysis and Design Technique, SofTech, 1976.
- Rumbaugh, J., Blaha, M., Premerlani, W., Frederick, E. and Lorensen, W., *Object-Oriented Modeling and Design*, Prentice-Hall, 1991.
- Senge, Peter M., *The Fifth Discipline*, Doubleday, 1990.
- Smith, Adam, *An Inquiry into the Wealth of Nations*, 1780, Thomas Dobson, 1796.
- Stewart III, G. Bennet, *Quest for Value*, Harper Collins, 1991.
- Toefler, Alvin, *Power Shift*, New York: Bantam Books, 1991.
- United States Air Force Project, ICAM Factory of the Future - IDEF0 Model, 1983.
- VA Electronic Health Record Modernization Functional Requirements VA118-17-R-2324 002A - VA Functional Requirements.pdf, 2017.
- Von Krogh, G., Ichijo, K., Nonaka, I., *Enabling Knowledge Creation,* Oxford Univ Press, 2000.
- WEF Global Competitiveness Report, www.weforum.org/reports/the-global-competitveness-report-2018, 2018.
- Wycoff, Joyce, *Mindmapping*, Berkley Books, 1991.

Record	Retention Period	Department
1] Market: Advertising		
Advertising agency files, artwork, copy, tear sheets	6 years	Advertising
Market research data, competitor files	Supersede	Marketing
Marketing programs	Active + 7 years	Marketing
Media / press kits / publicity photos/records	3 years	Marketing
Mailing lists	Active + 3 years	Communications
Donor, benefactor lists and records	Active + 3 years	Communications
Trade show, special event project files	3 years	Marketing
Publications, catalogs, price lists, contracts, correspondence records	Active + 6 years	Sales
Customer orders, rebate, co-op advertising payments, reports	Active + 6 years	Sales
Training materials	Active + 6 years	Sales
Press clippings and releases, slides and photographs, TV & radio transcripts	Active + 6 years	Public Relations
2] Develop: Research Records		
Institutional Review Board records: 1] IRB meeting minutes, records of continuing review activities 2] R&D proposals, scientific evaluations, consent documents, and progress reports; 3] Copies of correspondence between IRB, investigators and written procedures; 4] List of IRB member resumes and relationship to the institution.	Indefinitely	Human Research Protections Program
Institutional Review Board (IRB) Research Department Records	21 years	
Medical device records	10 yrs after date	Investigative Site
Patient/subject records relating to research, including consent forms	10 yrs after complete	Investigative Site
Records relating to allegations of research misconduct	10 years after report	Research Admin
Research-related financial records, supporting documents, statistical records, and all records pertinent to awards or receipt of monies to conduct a research study,	10 years after research completed	Grants Management Office/Research Service
3] Purchase		
RFQs/Vendor quotes/no bid	Active + 6 years	Purchasing
Purchase orders and contracts	Active + 6 years	Purchasing
Receiving and inspection report record	Active + 6 years	Purchasing
Requisitions and inventory records	Active + 6 years	Purchasing
Acknowledgements from vendor (after completion of job or contract)	Active +1year	Purchasing
Transfer purchase order	Active +1year	Purchasing
Packing slips from vendor	Active +1year	Purchasing
Receiving and inspection report record	Active +1year	Purchasing
Production schedules	Active +1year	Purchasing
Part releases	Active +1year	Purchasing
4] Deliver: QUALITY ASSURANCE / INFECTION CONTROL RECORDS		
Incident or occurrence reports	21 years	Dept of report/Risk
Infection control records (plus logs of incidents related to infections & communicable diseases)	21 years	Infection Control
Patient complaints	21 years	Quality/Patient Relations
QA/QI Plan	10 yrs after new plan	Quality
Quality, risk, utilization records (with minutes, departmental reports, reports to Board)	21 years	Quality
4] Deliver: CLINICAL& CLINICAL-RELATED RECORDS		
Patient Medical Records	Permanent	Medical Records
Statistical records (admissions, services, discharges, transfers, department statistics, daily census, outpatient department patient lists)	10 years	Administration
Tissue records -- Human tissue records (other than related to reproduction) intended for transplantation, artificial insemination, and implantation,	21 years	Departments for transplant, implant or insemination
Tracings EKG/EEG/EMG/Fetal Monitor; Cardiology/Radiology/Obstetrics-Gynecology	Adults: 10 years	Medical Records
Mammograms	21 years	Radiology
Orders (including the NPI of the physician ordering imaging service)	10 years	Radiology
Radiology or nuclear medicine films, scans & other images not medical records	21 years	Radiology
Immunohematology, blood and blood product, transfusion records	21 years	Hematology
Instrument records (plus printouts, worksheets, calibration, maintenance records)	10 years	Engineering
Lab reports, all other	21 years	Laboratory
Plasmaphereses records	21 years	Laboratory

Record	Retention Period	Department
Proficiency testing–related records	10 years	Laboratory
Syphilis serology reports	21 years	Laboratory
Requisitions	7 years	Laboratory
Fetal Monitoring Strips	21 years	Laboratory
Infection Control Reports	21 years	Laboratory
Pathology Slides, Reports & Records	21 years	Laboratory
Radiology or Nuclear Medicine	21 years	Laboratory
Films, Scans & Other Image Records	21 years	Laboratory
Records of tissue and nontransplant anatomic parts released for transplantation	21 years	Laboratory
Release or Disposal of Human Remains	21 years	Laboratory
Transfusion Records	21 years	Laboratory
4] Deliver: Laboratory, Pathology and Blood Services Records		
Accession records	10 years	Laboratory
Blood donation–related records.	21 years	Laboratory
Complaints regarding lab standards, including resulting investigations and corrective actions	10 years	Laboratory
Cytogenetics reports	25 years	Laboratory
Cytotechnologist work standards and related records	10 years	Laboratory
Equipment records (including preventative maintenance, service & repair records)	Active + 10 years	Laboratory
Histopathology, oral pathology and dermatopathology reports.	21 years	Laboratory
Bacteriology Slide (on which diagnosis depends)	3 years	Laboratory
Blood Film (a shorter period may be required due to storage size)	3 years	Laboratory
Bone Marrow Biopsy	21 years	Laboratory
Histopathology Block	21 years	Laboratory
Recipient Blood Specimens stoppered at 6 degrees Celsius	1 week	Laboratory
Requests for Cytogenetic Tests 7 years	7 years	Laboratory
All Other Lab Reports	21 years	Laboratory
4] Deliver: EMERGENCY ROOM & EMS		
Ambulance Patient Care Records	6 years	Emergency Room
Emergency Department (ED) Central Log of Patients	21 years	Emergency Room
Patient Transfer Records	21 years	Emergency Room
Daily Census/Outpatient Department Patient Lists	6 years	Emergency Room
ED Diversion Sheet	6 years	Emergency Room
Emergency Room (ER) List of On–Call Physicians	21 years	Emergency Room
Ambulance Corps Records Administrative	21 years	Emergency Room
4] Deliver: Clinical & Clinical-Related Records: Pharmacy Service Records		
Clinical notes made in the pharmacy's computer system	10 years	Pharmacy
Controlled substances records: transactions, requisitions, inventory, and disposal	10 years	Pharmacy/ Nursing
Orders / prescriptions for dispensed drugs	10 years[2]	Records/Pharmacy
5] Support: Records Specific to Physician Practice: Ambulatory Surgery Centers ("ASC") and Diagnostic & Treatment Centers (DTC)		
Admission, pre & post-surgical assessment & discharge records	10 years	ASC/DTC
Clinical records: consent forms, medical/drug history, immunization, medical orders, exam/diagnostic/tests reports, consultative findings, diagnosis, anesthesia, psychosocial assessment, referrals, progress note(s), follow-up plans, discharge)	10 years	ASC/DTC
Corporate records: list of directors, officers & members or stockholders of NGOs or business corporate operator and partnership operator, certificate of incorporation).	Permanent	ASC/DTC
Disclosure of physician financial interests or ownership in the Facility	10 years	ASC/DTC
List of surgical procedures	Permanent	ASC/DTC
Operating Room Register	Permanent	ASC/DTC
Records of grievances and complaints	21 years	ASC/DTC
Transfer agreements	10 yrs after terminated	ASC/DTC
5] Support: Records Specific to Skilled Nursing Homes Long Term Care Facilities		
Activity programs records: activities director resume, current roster of program resident participants and their participation at each activity for 12 previous months	6 years	Nursing Home
Bed hold records (including the Medicaid Patient/Resident Absence Register, Status of Bed Reservation Form, records verifying number and nature of bed reservations)	10 years	Nursing Home
Chronological list of admitted residents, by name, identifying data, place of transfer	10 years	Nursing Home
Chronological listing of residents discharged and reason, by name.	10 years	Nursing Home

Record	Retention Period	Department
All clinical records (including a record of the residents	10 years	Nursing Home
Daily census record	10 years	Nursing Home
Dietary service records	6 years	Nursing Home
Disaster and emergency preparedness plan	Permanent	Nursing Home
Feeding assistant training records	Employment+6 yrs	Nursing Home
Films, scans, and other image records	10 years	Nursing Home
Long Term Care Patient Assessment Forms	10 years	Nursing Home
Nursing service administration (including organization chart/master staffing plan)	Permanent	Nursing Home
Physician certification	10 years	Nursing Home
Resident non-medical record (including a general fiscal record for each resident)	10 years	Nursing Home
Specialized rehabilitative therapy service records.	6 years	Nursing Home
Transfer or affiliation agreements	10 years	Nursing Home
5] Support: RECORDS SPECIFIC TO HOME HEALTH AGENCIES		
Clinical records,	10 years	Home Health Agency
Corporate records specific to home health agencies	Permanent	Home Health Agency
List of personnel – Note: This must be retained at the branch office	10 years from list date	Home Health Agency
Patient rosters Note: This must be retained at the branch office	Permanent	Home Health Agency
Physicians' certifications and recertifications	10 years	Home Health Agency
Plan of care and comprehensive interdisciplinary patient assessment	10 years	Home Health Agency
Records of grievances, complaints and appeals	10 years	Home Health Agency
5] Support: RECORDS SPECIFIC TO HOSPICE		
Agreements with other facilities and/or individuals for out-/in- inpatient services	10 yrs	Hospice
Clinical records (including orders, physical exam, history, consents, notes, etc)	10 years	Hospice
Physician certification and recertification of terminal illness	7 years	Hospice
Plan of care and comprehensive assessment	7 years	Hospice
Corporate records specific to hospice operation	Permanent	Hospice
Patient / family rosters; Note: This must be retained at each hospice sub office	Permanent	Hospice
Records of grievances, complaints and appeals	21 years	Hospice
6] Manage Staff: EMPLOYMENT RECORDS		
Historical materials (pictures, publications, etc.)	Permanent	Communications
Newsletters (internal)	3 years	Communications
Speeches by corporate officers	Permanent	Communications
Affirmative Action plans	Active +10 years	Workforce Planning
COBRA notices	6 years	Benefits
Pension / 401(k) Retirement Plan, vesting files and related records	6 years from retiring	Benefits
Employee service & eligibility records (including hrs worked, breaks in service)	Permanent	Benefits
HIPAA forms	Permanent	Benefits
Group life plan – active employees, retirees	Active+6 years	Insurance
Long-term disability files	Active +6 years	Insurance
Incentives, awards	TAX+6 years	Compensation
Employee handbook (original)	Active +10 years	Staffing
Employee hazardous materials exposure records	Permanent	Staffing
Employee reference, background checks	Active +3 years	Staffing
Employee relocation, move records	6 years	Staffing
Personnel records (excluding medical records)	Employment + 6 yrs	Human Resources
Worker's Compensation records relating to injury/illness incurred by an employees	Date of injury+18 yrs	Risk
Personnel records for volunteers, students, or non-compensated personnel	6-10 years for records	Health Services/HR
Job descriptions	Superseded	Staffing
Job posting info (agency notices, advertising, correspondence)	3 years	Staffing
Class attendance records	Active +3 years	Training
Training manuals, videos	Active +3 years	Training
Application materials, employment inquiries, applications, resumes, and job orders	6 years from date	Human Resources
Collective bargaining agreements	6 years from last date	Human Resources
EEO forms and related records / recordings	6 years from filing	Human Resources
Employee Disability Plan and related records	6 yrs from termination	Human Resources
Employee medical records (as required by OSHA: occupational injury / illness)	30 yrs after employed	Employee Health Service
Employee training certifications	21 years	HRM/ Employee's dept
Employment contracts, benefits plans and related documents	10 years	HR / PAANS

Record	Retention Period	Department
Pay scales (including charts used for salary for job class & salary guidelines)	6 years	Human Resources
Employment testing, plus any exams considered connected with personnel action	6 years from action	Human Resources
FMLA authorized job protected leave records	6 yrs from terminated	Human Resources
I-9 Forms to validate legal status to work	6 yrs after employed	HR/ Employee's Dept
Notices of opportunities: e.g., ads, job openings, promotions, training, overtime	Active + 6 years	Human Resources
Paid time off records, including hospital or other 3rd party payer for leave	Tax filing+6 years	HR/ Payroll
Employment taxes and related documents (IRS forms W-2, W-4, W-9, 1099, 940, 941, returns filed and confirmation numbers, records benefits and reimbursement)	Tax filing+6 years	Human Resources
Payroll records (earnings records, hours worked, gross wages, deductions, net wages, wage rate tables, and time sheets with daily start/end times)	Employee term+6 yrs	HR/ Payroll
Personnel decisions / policies, hiring, promotion, demotion, transfer, training, layoff, recall, termination, merit and seniority systems	6 years from date of personnel action	Human Resources/ Employee's Department
6] Manage Staff: MEDICAL STAFF / RESIDENCY RECORDS		
Affiliation agreements (medical education, Residency and Fellowship programs)	10 yrs after terminate	Office Academic Affairs
Credentialing records (Medical Staff personnel records)	Active + 20 years	Credentialing/ PAANS
Disciplinary actions (involving Medical Staff members)	21 years	Medical Affairs/ Credentials
Patient complaints regarding care (involving Medical Staff members)	21 years	Quality/Credentialing/Risk
Personnel records (Medical Staff)	Active + 20 years	PAANS
Rejected applications (Medical Staff)	6 yrs from determine	Credentialing / Quality
Residency rotation agreements	10 yrs after terminate	Office Academic Affairs
7] Manage IT & Technology:		
Information technology governance documents	Permanent	
HIPAA privacy and security policies and procedures	Active + 6 years	IT
System upgrade reports	3 years	IT
Utilization and uptime reports	3 years	IT
Application manuals and user guide	3 years	IT
Applications curriculum and training manuals	3 years	IT
Taxonomy and Database documentation, web page programming	10 years	IT
Equipment Manuals and Maintenance guides	As long as in service	Engineering
Equipment utilization and failure reports	As long as in service	Engineering
8] FINANCE:		
Billing records, claims forms, charge slips, patient/debtor billing history, business and accounting claims records – Medicare Secondary Payor questionnaires	10 years	Finance
Correspondence, telephone logs regarding contact with govmnt representatives and/or billing agents, and commercial payers regarding billing-related issues	10 years	Managed Care/ Finance, Dept of correspondence
Donor records related to dedicated donor funds and special funds, correspondence	Permanent	Finance/ Foundation
Annual reports & financial statements	Permanent	Finance
Explanation of Benefits	10 years	Finance
Financial plan	Active +2 years	Budgets/Forecasts
Financial reports, including work papers and general ledgers	Current year + 6 yrs	Finance
Financial statements	Current year + 6 yrs	Finance
Procurement records: Bids (accepted/rejected)	Active + 7 years	Procurement
Procurement records: Purchase orders/supply requisitions (electronic, paper)	10 years	Procurement
Self-pay patient records, including attempts at collection	Current+6 years	Finance
Amortization records	6 years	Accts Payable
Cash disbursements	6 years	Accts Payable
Charitable contribution records	6 years	Accts Payable
Check registers / Paid check registers - monthly (ledgers)	6 years	Accts Payable
Cost sheets, statements, cost accounting records, cost reports	6 years	Accts Payable
Debit advises	6 years	Accts Payable
Expense reports (including travel expenses)	6 years	Accts Payable
Insurance payments (unemployment)	6 years	Accts Payable
Insurance payments (worker compensation)	6 years	Accts Payable
Invoices (original) - and check vouchers	6 years	Accts Payable
Mortgage payments	6 years	Accts Payable
Petty cash records	6 years	Accts Payable
Purchase order requisitions, registers	6 years	Accts Payable
Recurring payment files	6 years	Accts Payable

Record	Retention Period	Department
Vouchers	6 years	Accts Payable
Aging - monthly A/R aging trial balance	6 years	Accts Receivable
Collections correspondence	6 years	Accts Receivable
Credit advice	6 years	Accts Receivable
Credit investigation requests	Active+6 years	Accts Receivable
Invoice / bills with back-up (Sales receipts)	6 years	Accts Receivable
Ledger vouchers - employees, general, city, tenants, advance	6 years	Accts Receivable
Budget forecasts (5 year)	Active+5 years	Budgets/Forecasts
Budgets, worksheets	Active+2 years	Budgets/Forecasts
Forecasts (1 year)	Active+2 years	Budgets/Forecasts
Bank deposits, slips, reconciliation, statements, facility activity	6 years	Cash
Capital asset records	Active+6 years	Cash
Cash receipts, books, journals, sales slips	6 years	Cash
Check copies (cancelled, returned)	6 years	Cash
Deposit slips	6 years	Cash
Acquisition cost records	Active+6 years	Financial Reports
Audit reports (external/internal)	6 years	Financial Reports
Audit workpaper package (annual)	6 years	Financial Reports
Client Contract File	Active+6 years	Financial Reports
Labor summary	3 years	Financial Reports
Management Reports	Active	Financial Reports
Profit / loss statements / reports	10 years	Financial Reports
Personnel Transaction Form (PTF) processing	6 years	Financial Reports
Securities SEC filings	Active+6 years	Financial Reports
Surveys - census bureau, government	6 years	Financial Reports
Balance sheets	6 years	General Ledger
Chart of accounts	6 years	General Ledger
Fixed asset ledgers (year-end run)	Active+6 years	General Ledger
General journals, postings, ledgers, control media	6 years	General Ledger
General ledger detail trial balances, monthly, annual	6 years	General Ledger
Depreciation schedules	Active+6 years	Journal Entries
Journal entries	6 years	Journal Entries
Sold property records	6 years	Journal Entries
Billing overage invoices	6 years	Lease Management
Equipment detail reports	Supersede	Lease Management
Non-labor reports	6 years	Lease Management
Assignments, attachments, garnishments	6 years	Payroll
Employee deduction authorizations	6 years	Payroll
Employee earnings records	6 years	Payroll
Flash Reports	6 years	Payroll
Invoices for temporary labor	6 years	Payroll
Registers (gross, net), off-cycle check updates	6 years	Payroll
Tax returns, filings - payroll	6 years	Payroll
Tax returns, filings - Social Security	6 years	Payroll
Tax workpapers - Social Security	6 years	Payroll
Time cards/sheets, attendance reports, sign-in/out sheets	6 years	Payroll
Unclaimed wage reports	6 years	Payroll
Protests, appeals, claims for refund	6 years	Tax
Research files	Supersede	Tax
Returns, filings, receipts, bills - federal , foreign, payroll, sales, state	6 years	Tax
State, local sales & use licenses	6 years	Tax
Work papers (operating division copies)	6 years	Tax
Cash packets	6 years	Treasury
Credit establishment letters, applications	Active+6 years	Treasury
Loan applications, agreements	Active+6 years	Treasury
Mortgage records (excluding agreement)	Active+6 years	Treasury
Wire transfers	6 years	Treasury
9] Manage Property: REAL ESTATE / LEASES		

Record	Retention Period	Department
Construction documents; blueprints	While hospital has title	Facilities/Real Estate
Deeds and titles to real property, right–of–way, correspondence	While hospital has title	Facilities/Real Estate
Leases/mortgages and agreements pertaining to ownership of land, buildings, fixtures or equipment	10 years	Facilities/Real Estate
Building layout, improvement plans, contracts (purchase, sale, lease)	Active+6 years	Facilities/ Engineering
Emergency action plans; Disaster recovery plans	Active+10 years	Facilities/ Engineering
Equipment logs	Superseded	Facilities/ Engineering
Lease abstracts	Active+10 years	Facilities/ Engineering
Maintenance/Repair records	Active+3years	Facilities/ Engineering
Property inventory	Superseded	Facilities/ Engineering
Real estate records	Permanent	Facilities/ Engineering
Building easements, water rights information	Permanent	Real Estate
Building zoning permits	Active + 3 years	Real Estate
Credit agreements, loan, financing, commitments, promissory notes	Active + 6 years	Real Estate
Partnership, joint venture agreements	Active + 6 years	Real Estate
Property deeds	Permanent	Real Estate
10] Manage Health/Safety: ENVIRONMENTAL / EQUIPMENT / SAFETY RECORDS		
Autoclave–related records (operation plan modification, time records: validation and challenge testing, protocols and test results; routine system's monitoring)	6 years	Engineering
Central supply services records and tests (including maintaining and recording time and temperature for each sterilization cycle and aeration cycle)	At least one year	Engineering
Equipment testing, maintenance and calibration records	21 years	Engineering
Fire protection records (preventative maintenance, and fire investigations)	6 years	Engineering
Material Safety Data Sheets (MSDS) and toxic substance use	30 years	Environmental
Occupational noise exposure related records, noise exposure	2 yrs	Engineering
OSHA required employee exposure records	Employment+ 0 years	Engineering
Radioisotopes–related records (including records of receipt, transfer, disposal)	3 yrs after transfer	Radiation Safety
Regulated medical waste–related records	6 years	Environmental
10] Manage Health/Safety: Risk Management Records		
Audit, adjustments	Active + 6 years	Insurance
Certificates to company (general, liability)	Permanent	Insurance
Claims – first & 3rd party liability (medical records, injury documentation, etc)	Active + 6 years	Insurance
Claims – release / settlements	Active + 6 years	Insurance
Insurance policies (general, liability)	Permanent	Insurance
Journal entry support data	TAX + 6 years	Insurance
Loss runs, summaries (annual)	Active + 6 years	Insurance
Certificates of Completion of Infection Control & Barrier Precaution Training	21 years	Security
Fire Protection	6 years	Security
Health & Safety Audiometric Test Record & Emergency Action Plans	Active + 30 years	Security
Health & Safety Hazardous Employee Exposure	Active + 30 years	Insurance
Health & Safety Illness, Injury, or Accident Reports (OSHA Form 301)	Active + 30 years	Insurance
Health & Safety Noise Exposure Measurements	Active + 30 years	Insurance
Material Safety Data Sheets	Active + 30 years	Insurance
11] Manage Legal and External Relationships: CONTRACTS		
Incident reports	3 years	Security
Log reports/ Visitor badge lists/ Visitor registration logs	3 years	Security
Contracts with health care providers / referral sources	10 yrs > termination	Contracting Department
Government contracts (correspondence, reports and contracts)	10 yrs after payment	Finance
Managed care contracts (including all fiscal and related administrative records)	10 yrs > termination	Managed Care
Litigation: Final Judgments, Settlements, and Court Orders	20 years	Legal
Insurance: policies/riders/certificates/papers	Permanent	Risk
Fidelity, surety bonds	Active + 6 years	Corporate
Foreign qualifications & related records	Permanent	Corporate
Investments – bonds, future, options, stock	TAX+6 years	Corporate
Proxies (including election of directors)	1 year	Corporate
Stock certificates, sales, transfers, ledgers, other records	Permanent	Corporate
Stockholder listings, records (notices, meetings, proxies)	Permanent	Corporate
Claims	Active + 6 years	Litigation

Record	Retention Period	Department
Subpoenas	6 years	Records of Department
Collections litigation files	Active + 6 years	Litigation
Memoranda & opinions	Active +10 years	Miscellaneous
Case files (pleadings, discovery, deposition, settlements)	Active + 6 years	Litigation
Contracts, licenses and related correspondence and documents	Active + 6 years	Contract
General business permits	Active + 3 years	Contract
11] Manage Legal and External Relationships: Reports to Department of Health		
Registers of admissions/discharges, births, deaths and surgical procedures	Permanent	Admit Medical Records
Reports of hospital-acquired infections and diseases and conditions	Permanent	Quality
Reports of suspected child abuse or neglect	10 years	Social Work/ Department
11] Manage Legal and External Relationships: INTELLECTUAL PROPERTY [12]		
Patents and patent applications and invention forms	Permanent	Intellectual Property
Trademark documents, assignment forms, correspondence	Active + 6 years	Intellectual Property
Royalty payments and patent agreements	Permanent	Intellectual Property
Laboratory and invention notebooks	Permanent	Legal Department
Outside submission of new product (drug) ideas	Permanent	Legal Department
Letters pertaining to patents, copyright and licensing agreements	Permanent	Legal Department
Results of double tests and regulatory (FDA) reporting	Permanent	Legal Department
Approvals and certifications	Permanent	Legal Department
12] Develop/manage business capabilities: Corporate / Administration / Legal		
By-Laws, Corporate and Medical Staff	Permanent	Legal
Certificates of Incorporation (including amendments)	Permanent	Legal
Certificates of Need	Permanent	Planning
Corporate Integrity Agreements	6 years	Compliance
Company policies & procedures manual (original)	Active+10 years	General
Corporate reorganizations	10 years	Corporate
Corporate voting records	Permanent	Corporate
Corporate acquisition, merger, divestiture records	10 years	Corporate
Corporate board of directors meeting notices	Permanent	Corporate
Corporate charters, by-laws, amendments, seals, incorporation records	Permanent	Corporate
Dividend records	6 years	Corporate
Filings: Governmental and Regulatory	Permanent	Department filing
Governmental Audits and Investigations (Federal and State)	15 years	Finance
IRS Letter Recognizing Tax-Exempt Status	Permanent	Finance
Licensing and accreditation surveys, inspections reports	Permanent	Quality
Meeting Minutes: Board of Trustees Committee and Departmental	Permanent	Body conducting meeting
Operating Certificates, Licenses, and Permits	Permanent	Planning
General Records Applicable to All Depts		
Company policies & procedures (correspondence explaining, but not establishing policy)	3 years	General
Complaint correspondence	3 years	General
General correspondence, chronology, reader files, correspondence calendars	3 years	General
Meeting plans & minutes	3 years	General
Organization charts	3 years	General
Trade association materials	3 years	General
12] Develop/manage business capabilities: RECORDS ADMINISTRATION		
Destruction reports, management procedures, transfer forms, Retention schedule	Permanent	Records Department
Retrieval requests, Vital records program/log	Permanent	Records Department

Note: These records do not need to be maintained for a specified t i m e period: (1) health insurance claims records maintained separately from employer's medical program and its records; (2) first aid records not involving medical treatment, loss of consciousness, restriction of work, or transfer to another job, if made on-site by a non-physician and if maintained separately from the employer's medical program and its records; and (3) Medical records of employees who have worked for less than one year need not be retained beyond the term of employment if they are provided to the employee upon the termination. For pharmacies doing Medicare Part D business, CMS expects Part D plans will require their pharmacies to maintain prescription records in their original format for the greater of 3 years or the period required by State law, and permit the records to be transferred to an electronic format that replicates the original prescription (such as a digitized image) for the remaining years of the 10-year Part D retention period. CMS Part D FAQ 14July2005 (ID:5137).

Define	Patient: regimen, required knowledge, behaviors, diet, exercise (Policy, Governance, Process, EHR)						Patient Value
Measure	Well-being: test, imaging, outcomes, records, compliance (Balance Scorecard)						
Analyze	Medical consult: Alternate treatments, drugs, R&D (office, hospital, transport, home, remote)						
Improve	Medical environment: knowledge, process, skills, technology, culture, drugs, systems (IoT, IT, HRM, Assets)						
Control	Manage: Compliance ⟩ Market ⟩ Develop ⟩ Purchase ⟩ *Deliver* ⟩ *Maintain* ⟩						

6σ	1.0 Initiate Treatment	2.0 Administer records	3.0 Diagnose	4.0 Intervene (IPU)	5.0 Rehabilitate	6.0 Provide custodial care
	1.1 Assure EMS Capability	& documents	3.1 Assess symptoms	4.1 Initiate IPU project	5.1 Initiate rehab project	6.1 Provide disability housing
	1.2 Respond to request	2.1 Register patient for care	3.2 Order tests	4.2 Administer drugs	5.2 Assure well-being	6.2 Provide non-medical service
	1.2 Mitigate symptoms	2.2 Document Diagnosis (SOAP)	3.3 Interpret cause	4.3 Execute IPU project	5.3 Perform rehab therapy	6.3 Provide food, medications & personal care
	1.3 Transport person	2.3 Record (intervention	3.4 Propose treatment	4.4 Audit IPU Result	5.4 Assess rehab progress	6.4 Provide nursing & (virtual) medical services
	1.4 Intervene in ER	& rehab) action	3.5 Plan treatment	4.5 Plan rehab	5.5 Verify patient wellness	6.5 Provide adapted transportation
Porter	1.5 Transfer or Release	2.4 Assure quality records	(Prepare Patient)			6.6 Assure I of T for medical devices
Revised		2.5 Record discharge of patient				

	Repository Taxonomy	Project Model	Tollgate Review Model	Collaboration Model		Health Outcomes Per unit cost
	⟩ Technology ⟩ HRM ⟩ Finance ⟩ Facilities ⟩ Legal ⟩					
	⟩ Audit ⟩ Direct ⟩ Adjust ⟩ Lead ⟩ Enable ⟩					

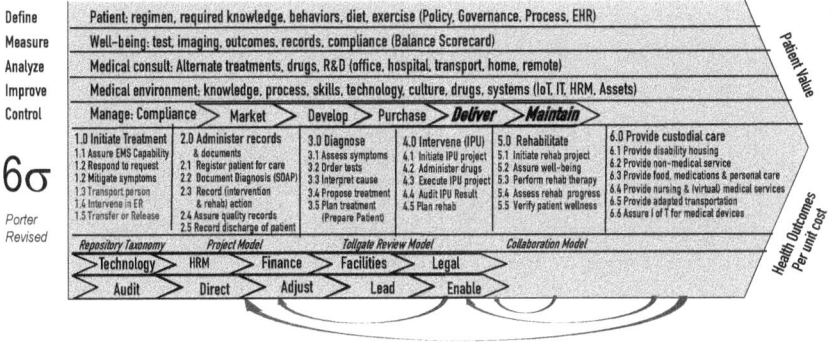

FEO Care for Patient

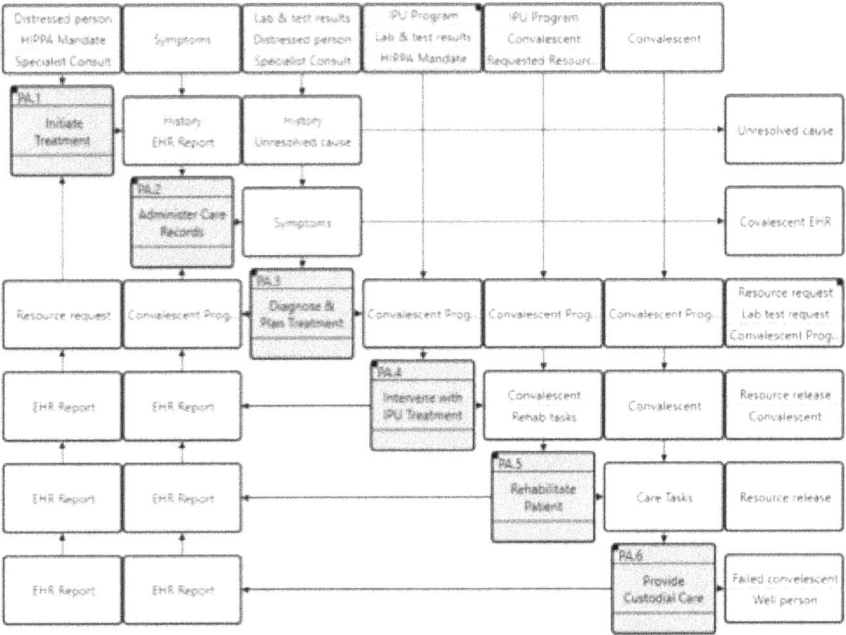

A0 Care for Patient Model

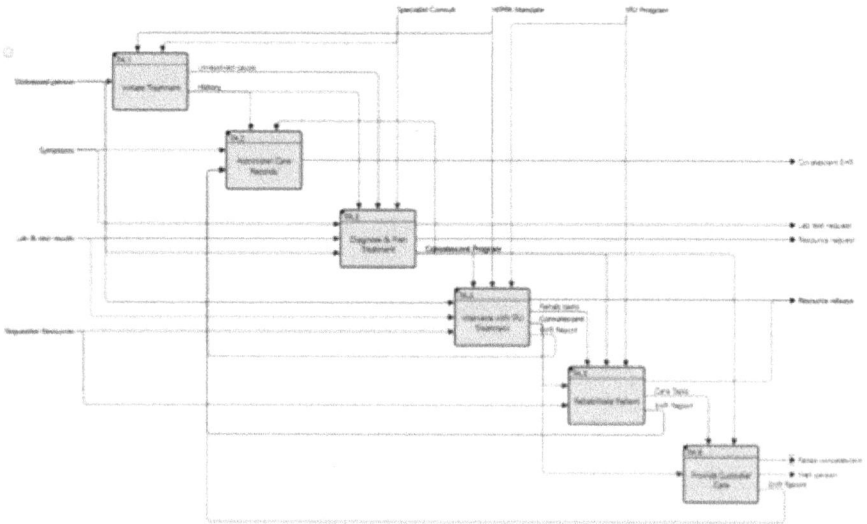

A-1 Initiate Treatment

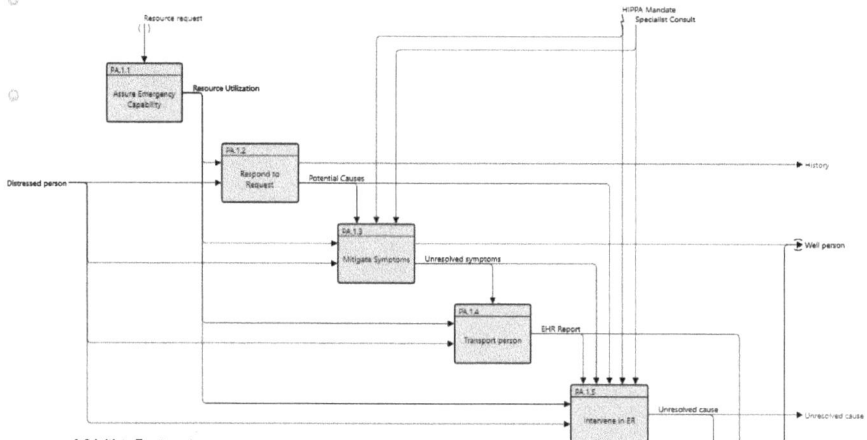

1.0 Initiate Treatment
1.1 Assure EMS Capability
1.2 Respond to request
1.3 Mitigate symptoms
1.4 Transport person
1.5 Intervene in ER
1.6 Transfer or Release

A-2 Administer Records & Documents

2.0 Administer records & documents
2.1 Register patient for care
2.2 Document Diagnosis (SOAP)
2.3 Record (intervention & rehab) action
2.4 Assure quality records
2.5 Record discharge of patient

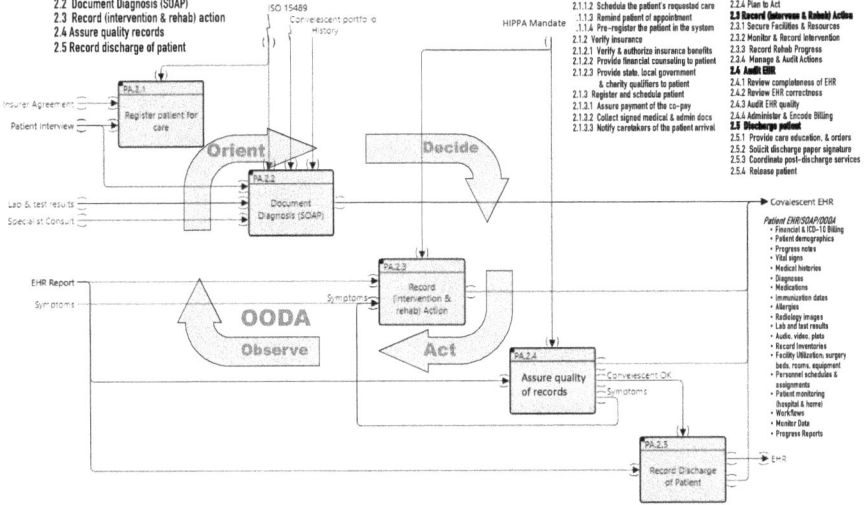

ISO 15489
Convalescent portfolio
History

HIPPA Mandate

2 Administer Care and Records
2.1 Receive the patient for care
2.1.1 Register Patient
2.1.1.1 Solicit referral source from the Patient
2.1.1.2 Schedule the patient's requested care
.1.1.2 Remind patient of appointment
.1.1.4 Pre-register the patient in the system
2.1.2 Verify insurance
2.1.2.1 Verify & authorize insurance benefits
2.1.2.2 Provide financial counseling to patient
2.1.2.3 Provide state, local government
  & charity qualifiers to patient
2.1.3 Register and schedule patient
2.1.3.1 Assure payment of the co-pay
2.1.3.2 Collect signed medical & admin docs
2.1.3.3 Notify caretakers of the patient arrival

2.2 Document Diagnosis (SOAP)
2.2.1 Observe (Subject)
2.2.2 Orient (Object)
2.2.3 Decide (Assess)
2.2.4 Plan to Act

2.3 Record (Intervene & Rehab) Action
2.3.1 Secure Facilities & Resources
2.3.2 Monitor & Record Intervention
2.3.3 Record Rehab Progress
2.3.4 Manage & Audit Actions

2.4 Audit EHR
2.4.1 Review completeness of EHR
2.4.2 Review EHR correctness
2.4.3 Audit EHR quality
2.4.4 Administer & Encode Billing

2.5 Discharge patient
2.5.1 Provide care education, & orders
2.5.2 Solicit discharge paper signature
2.5.3 Coordinate post-discharge services
2.5.4 Release patient

Insurer Agreement
Patient Interview

PA.2.1
Register patient for care

Orient

Decide

PA.2.2
Document Diagnosis (SOAP)

Lab & test results
Special st Consult

EHR Report
Symptoms

PA.2.3
Record (Intervention & rehab) Action

Symptoms

OODA

Observe

Act

PA.2.4
Assure quality of records

Convalescent OK
Symptoms

PA.2.5
Record Discharge of Patient

Convalescent EHR

Patient EHR/SOAP/OODA
· Financial & ICD-10 Billing
· Patient demographics
· Progress notes
· Vital signs
· Medical histories
· Diagnoses
· Medications
· Immunization dates
· Allergies
· Radiology images
· Lab and test results
· Audio, video, plots
· Record inventories
· Facility Utilization, surgery
  beds, rooms, equipment
· Personnel schedules &
  assignments
· Patient monitoring
  (hospital & home)
· Workflows
· Monitor Data
· Progress Reports

EHR

A3 Diagnose & Plan Care

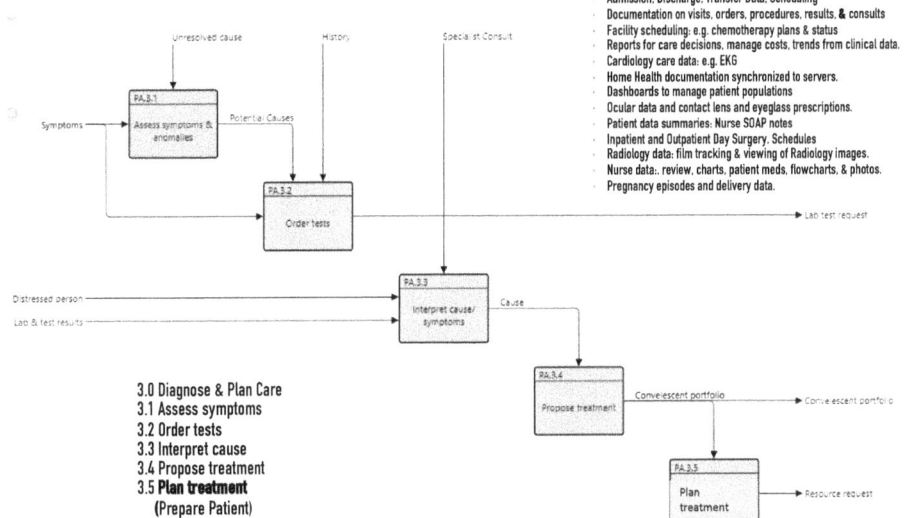

· ER visits: occupied rooms, room and bed status.
· Admission, Discharge, Transfer Data, Scheduling
· Documentation on visits, orders, procedures, results, & consults
· Facility scheduling: e.g. chemotherapy plans & status
· Reports for care decisions, manage costs, trends from clinical data.
· Cardiology care data: e.g. EKG
· Home Health documentation synchronized to servers.
· Dashboards to manage patient populations
· Ocular data and contact lens and eyeglass prescriptions.
· Patient data summaries: Nurse SOAP notes
· Inpatient and Outpatient Day Surgery. Schedules
· Radiology data: film tracking & viewing of Radiology images.
· Nurse data:. review, charts, patient meds, flowcharts, & photos.
· Pregnancy episodes and delivery data.

Unresolved cause
History
Specialist Consult

PA.3.1
Assess symptoms & anomalies

Symptoms
Potential Causes

PA.3.2
Order tests

Lab test request

Distressed person
Lab & test results

PA.3.3
Interpret cause/ symptoms

Cause

3.0 Diagnose & Plan Care
3.1 Assess symptoms
3.2 Order tests
3.3 Interpret cause
3.4 Propose treatment
3.5 **Plan treatment**
  (Prepare Patient)

PA.3.4
Propose treatment

Convalescent portfolio
Convalescent portfolio

PA.3.5
Plan treatment

Resource request

A-4 Intervene with Treatment

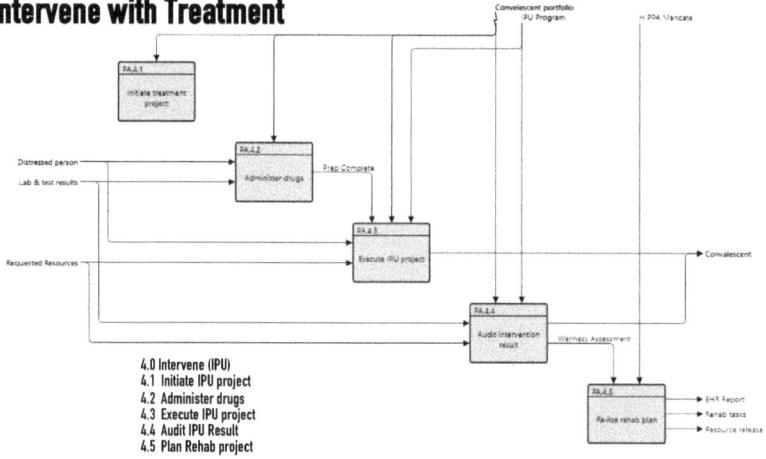

4.0 Intervene (IPU)
4.1 Initiate IPU project
4.2 Administer drugs
4.3 Execute IPU project
4.4 Audit IPU Result
4.5 Plan Rehab project

A-5 Rehabilitate

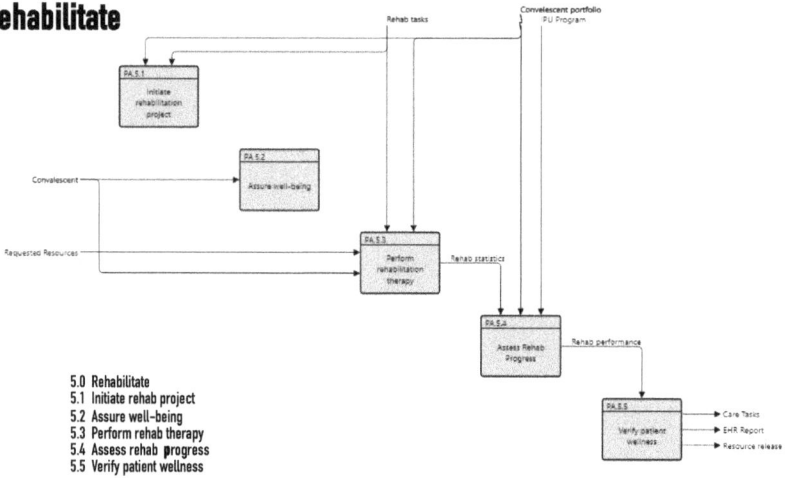

5.0 Rehabilitate
5.1 Initiate rehab project
5.2 Assure well-being
5.3 Perform rehab therapy
5.4 Assess rehab progress
5.5 Verify patient wellness

A-6 Provide Custodial Care

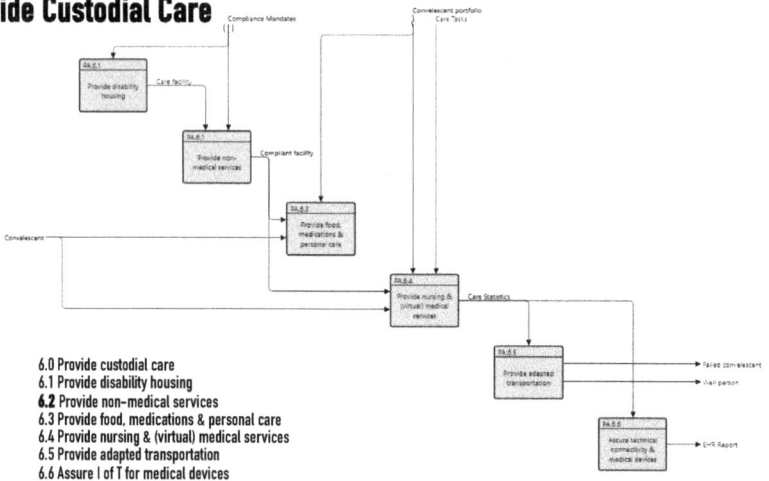

6.0 Provide custodial care
6.1 Provide disability housing
6.2 Provide non-medical services
6.3 Provide food, medications & personal care
6.4 Provide nursing & (virtual) medical services
6.5 Provide adapted transportation
6.6 Assure I of T for medical devices

Hospital's current price gouging will soon bankrupt the USA. Healthcare is $4.1 TRILLION (20% of GDP) and climbing. In a centuries old medical tradition, doctors charge rich people enough to cover poor people's treatment. Good insurance now equals rich. 190 million people in the USA have private health care. Insurers protect us from price gouging hospitals, but constant renegotiation adds significant expense. Insurers getting 20% for administration seems exorbitant, but pales in comparison to 500% hospital mark ups. Legislation has been inadequate: "Hospital list prices are set at exorbitant levels to extract higher reimbursements from insurance companies. ....no one knowledgeable about billing would agree to pay [hospital's listed prices]." (thehill.com/opinion/healthcare/414294-congress-should-broaden-legislation-to-curb-medical-price-gouging)

SOAP note (Subjective, Objective, Assessment, Plan) documents the way health care providers write notes in a patient's chart.

What follows is a SOAP note to fix for USA healthcare.

Subject Component documents the Chief Complaint (CC)

1] USA healthcare expenditures are 20% of GDP; $4.1 trillion.

2] 5% of the population accounts for 50% of medical expenditures.

3] 30 million people have no insurance.

4] Many rural and remote communities have inadequate healthcare.

5] Bills to patients are usually between 2 to 23 times actual cost.

6] USA drug prices are 30% higher than in Europe.

7] Medical debt puts 20% of Americans into bankruptcy.

8] Medical error may be the leading cause of death in the USA.

9] All legislation continues to not "fix" these problems.

Objective Component documents information from observations and interpretation of cause from symptoms.

1] Patients sign an agreement to pay all bills with no knowledge of cost until after treatment leaving them no recourse to gouging.

2] Operating cost of many medical facilities is more than can be reasonably billed to its patients resulting in gouging or poor care.

3] Some medical staff regularly perform unnecessary procedures.

4] High medical usage patients include seniors with multiple maladies and patients with chronic conditions or drug addictions.

5] Outcomes are poorly measured for diagnosis/intervention/rehab.

6] Insurers and medical facilities are inappropriately regulated.

7] Remote area infrastructure is inadequate to support telemedicine.

8] Telemedical consult invoices are sometimes denied by insurers.

Assessment Component documents a (medical) diagnosis.

Congress must pass legislation to require:

1] CMS to publish a recommended and standard average price list with standard DRGs and WHO coded items.

2] Medical facilities must publish their price for the same items.

3] All insurance will be in a Medicare framework varying only in deductible/copay based on age/gender/health.

4] All medical facilities and insurance companies to become ISO 9001 compliant to assure quality and transparency of process.

5] Health care providers to revise their patient payment contact to read: "I, <patient>, agree to pay for treatment in billing that is not more than <xx>% over the CMS standard prices."

6] All disputes go to binding arbitration with payout maximums.

7] Big Pharma offers best drug price relative to foreign contracts.

Plan Component documents treatment of USA Healthcare system.

Step 1] Regulate the healthcare and insurance markets effectively:

- Employers may purchase group base and supplemental plans for their employees in a Medicare insurance framework.
- Insurers can offer family plans where each family member may have different deductibles and copays.
- Community programs will provide free exams, promote healthy behaviors, and coordinate with social programs.
- High Usage/Risk Pool (>$500K in medical costs qualifies) to provide stringent oversight for high medical service use/abuse.
- CMS will partially fund HURP insurance pools for private insurers to reduce the risk for other group insurers.
- Malpractice and/or excessive billing claims go to arbitration.
- All healthcare facilities and insurers must be ISO9001 certified.
- Initiate a national telemedicine program with adequate telecom.

Step 2] Create a proof-of-concept model that delivers integrated, transparent, accountable healthcare.

- Penalize any healthcare facility or insurer that fails to be ISO 9001 compliant and properly publish prices (transparency).
- Provide a policy and procedure manual for a region leveraging telemedicine to integrate EMS, medical facilities and social services and specify a regional disaster plan.
- Institute a community paramedic program performed in the home by EMS personnel to assure Advanced Life Support EMS everywhere.
- Provide Community Paramedic and Physician Assistant certification education for nurses and EMTs.
- Insure major hospitals have ER staff and telemedicine to support rural (remote) healthcare in their region.
- Make major hospital support systems available to the region (e.g., EHR, IT, finance, HR, ERM).

- Develop elder-driven care plans based on quality-of-life goals.
- Assist elders and their family caregivers to get in-home support.

Step 3] Use CMS[1] insurance regions plus one to transition to single payer private insurance and healthcare.

- There will be one insurance policy framework, Medicare with its supplements and variants adopted from Obamacare as follows:
- Bronze= Medicare: $1000 Deductible/40% Copay.
- Silver= Medicare: $500 Deductible/30% Copay.
- Gold = Medicare (after age 65): $200 Deductible/20% Copay.
- Platinum = Veteran; No Pay.
- CMS will issue an RFP for one MAC to insure HURP with Federal government subsidies in the USA.
- CMS will issue an RFP for insurers as MACs to bid a fixed price for one insurer to provide Medicare in a CMS region.
- CMS will provide a Business Plan template to guide non-profit regional insurance organization start-ups.
- CMS pays MACs monthly negotiating overrun compensation.
- Insurers offer supplemental plans: prices may vary with age, gender, lifestyle, previous usage, and preconditions.
- Subsidies for the poor are provided as defined in Obamacare.
- CHIPS and IHS would be modified to qualify under Medicaid.

Step 4] Transition the Federal government from providing healthcare to regulating, paying and auditing insurers:

- Require all MACs, insurers and medical facilities to be ISO 9001 (or ISO 13485-medical device) certified by the FDA.
- Privatize VA, DOD and Indian medical facilities: sell facilities but, require services unique to its community.
- Hospitals bill CMS (MACs) and supplemental insurers with FDA audits.
- Insurers negotiate payments to hospitals from supplemental insurance premiums and Medicare.
- Patients pay the remainder based on their deductibles/copays and supplemental insurance agreement.
- As hospital service costs decline, MACs can lower deductibles and copays.

---

[1] *A Medicare Administrative Contractor (MAC) is a private health care insurer that has been awarded a contract to administer multi-state Medicare claims in one of ten geographic jurisdictions.*

MAC activities include:

- *Process and make Medicare FFS payments*
- *Enroll providers in Medicare*
- *Handle provider reimbursement services*
- *Audit institutional provider cost reports*
- *Handle redetermination requests (1st stage appeals process)*
- *Respond to provider inquiries*
- *Educate providers about Medicare FFS billing requirements*
- *Establish local coverage determinations (LCD's)*
- *Review medical records for selected claims*
- *Coordinate with CMS and other FFS contractors*

Abstract

A philosophy of engineering is needed to derive a new engineering body of knowledge and the governance practices to create sustainable artifacts and audit the use of AI on all digital platforms (e.g. planes, cars, trucks farm and construction equipment as well as the Internet), particularly those elements that cause societal harm by misrepresenting facts or misinterpreting the environment.

A global discourse should be based on a Philosophy of Engineering facilitated by modeling knowledge flow to value and system engineering as fundamental to understanding the creation and auditing of sustainable artifacts and AI systems. It is important to understand that most complex systems are digital platforms with a significant AI component. Two Boeing Plane crashes were caused by two properly functioning AI components that communicated improperly with each other. Since 1994, 70 million automotive vehicles were infected with software issues.

This paper examines the requirements for a philosophy of engineering necessary to derive a new engineering body of knowledge and the governance practices needed to oversee all AI platforms, particularly those elements that cause societal harm by posing a risk to life, safety, health, welfare, or governance of its citizens.
Keywords: philosophy, knowledge, flow, value, AI, artifacts

I Introduction

The pervasiveness of AI, digital platforms and social media makes them a battleground for bad actors to hack AI controlled artifacts as well as fabricate and propagate massive amounts of harmful information, such as hate speech, discrimination, violent extremism, child sexual abuse, disinformation and misinformation, with massive online engagement. There is an urgent need for broad collaborations among various stakeholders, including academia researchers from multi-disciplines, technologists, law and policy makers, non-profit organizations, private sectors, end users and most importantly, engineers. To begin this collaboration some essential philosophical foundations and governance practices are needed.

In her book Harvard Sociology Professor Shoshana Zuboff asserts that the fundamental construct of social order in our information civilization is controlled by the surveillance capitalist giants– Apple, Microsoft, Amazon, Google/Alphabet, Facebook/Meta though they were never elected to govern. These corporations constitute a sweeping political-economic information oligopoly which is now aided by artificial intelligence (AI) and that migrates across sectors and economies. Democratic and authoritarian governments alike depend on it for population-scale extraction of human-generated data, computation, prediction, and oppression.

At the center of the enabling capability are the social platforms, the breeding grounds for increasingly alarming practices that assault individual dignity and social harmony. They have escalated the scale and severity of social threats in the communication, notably amplifying issues such as misinformation, disinformation, and fake news, alongside exacerbating hate speech and ideological, as well as political, polarization.

The World Economic Forum rates misinformation and disinformation as the #1 global threat in 2024.

Significant as this is, it misses thee critical issue that all complex artifacts are also now digital platforms, enabled by AI, that could be hacked or misused. This includes vehicles of all types and military artifacts.

Two Boeing 737 MAX airliners crashed, one in 2018 and again in 2019, killing hundreds. Investigations are looking at the way two properly functioning AI components communicated improperly with each other. In one of the crashes, a pilot-autopilot struggle appears to have happened 21 times before the aircraft crashed into the sea. Information so far suggests a situation where inadequate testing and rushed practices led to some of these real disasters.

According to Wards, "Since [1994], more than 1,000 software-related recalls have occurred, potentially affecting 70.1 million vehicles." From this it appears that software is being used to correct mechanical problems in vehicles rather than finding ways of fixing the mechanical problems.

New knowledge has been used by engineers to create artifacts at a rate that is precipitating a decline in confidence of society's administrative functions, institutions, and leadership. It is caused in part by ubiquitous access to the harmful content and bad behavior on the Internet and elsewhere with unaudited use of AI platforms. Furthermore, engineered artifacts have contributed to these crises by pandering to people's decadent and the military's lethal wishes. Key to assuring societies' sustainability is for engineers to productively begin to engage in a global discourse.

Zuboff asks these additional questions: What may be known? Who knows? Who decides who knows? Who decides who decides who knows? What knowledge is produced? How is that knowledge distributed? What authority governs that distribution? What power sustains that authority?

The answer is: no one is being held accountable.

Engineered artifacts have contributed to societal crises by pandering to people's every decadent wish: Internet, media, microprocessor guided cars, phones, boats, transport, ATVs, entertainment, guns, etc. and support the military with lethal weapons.

Who can ultimately fix it? Not lawyers, doctors, writers, politicians, artists, social workers, activists, or managers, but mostly engineers. Specifically, engineers in an independent industry association with a relationship to engineering communities and academic institutions. An agile independent body is a key element to establishing standards and standard processes for the regulation necessary to address the associated risks and make sure we can all trust the information and platforms we are using.

Key to assuring societies' sustainability and resolving the current crises presented by social platforms is for engineers to productively engage in a global discourse especially on critical issues that support societal, economic, and ecological sustainability. This may help prevent governments and activists' initiatives 'unintended consequences' from the uses of platforms often based on simplified, local views of reality. To this end, value discussions need to be guided more by rationality, ethics, and sustainable alternatives rather than just by profit, power, recreation, comfort, cost, security, hysteria, and activism.

This paper presents an overview of a systems engineering approach to resolving the harmful aspects of AI driven artifacts and social platforms from an extensive view of philosophy, knowledge, flow, value, and novelty, which can be used to provide solutions to building artifacts and resolving anomalies. It argues that an engineering philosophy can be a guide to reframing the problem and going beyond existing knowledge to promote a system and discipline constrained by moral guidance and a more comprehensive view of value to:
- Filter knowledge (truth) from Internet nonsense,
- Precipitate and validate innovation and novelty to benefit individual well-being,
- Increase participation in defining solutions for societal value and ecological sustainability,
- Provide a foundation for creation of high-value artifacts.

II Philosophers

The following is a brief account of some philosophy and a few philosophers who can provide perspective to engineers that audit, govern and manage the next horizon of digital platforms.

Jürgen Habermas, in his book, *Legitimation Crisis*, claims as societies evolve, they are in danger of entering a state of crisis; crises arise when the structure of a social system cannot solve the problems required for its continued existence. These crises are not produced by external changes, but through internal incompatible system-imperatives that cannot be integrated. Crises disintegrate societies when their members feel their social identity is threatened. He defines:
- Social integration as related to the systems of institutions in which people are socially interrelated;
- System integration as related to institutions with steering performances of self-regulated systems;
- Social systems as life-worlds that are symbolically structured and maintain their boundaries and continued existence by mastering or obfuscating (possibly using AI) the complexity of a changing environment.

In modern capitalistic societies, political systems are subordinate to the socio-cultural and economic systems:
- Socio-cultural subsystems have standard structures that include a status system and sub-cultural forms of life with underlying categories that include distribution of privately available rewards and rights of disposition.
- Political subsystems have standard structures that include political institutions (state) with underlying categories that include distribution of legitimate power and available organizational rationality.
- Economic subsystems have standard structures that include economic institutions (relations of production) with underlying categories that include distribution of economic power and available forces of production.

Martin Heidegger defines 'enframing' as seeing everything as a framework of means, ends, causes, and effects. He claims technological thinking confuses us by 'revealing' everything to us as a resource available and as a means to an end where human thinking (or AI) is not able to solve problems presented by technology, explaining the decline of society's confidence in administrative functions (e.g. government), which is one contemporary consequence of the widespread use of social platforms. Heidegger believes that "even if a god is taken as a secularized notion of the sacred..." it provides the basis for faith in society's institutions and functions even if we are not confident in them and even if we do not believe in God.

Alfred North Whitehead answers the requirement for a secular god and provides a way to bolster our faith in institutions and leadership. Combining concepts of Eastern and Western philosophy, Whitehead's god's primordial and consequent nature supports his explanation of 'reality' as process, helping us to see a way to become more confident in how the engineered world works. Eastern philosophers assert all intellectual disciplines must embrace the Absolute in order to precipitate novelty that could be used to engineer innovative support for the world's societies.

Carl Sanders Peirce claims support this perspective, and to the processes of induction and deduction, must be added the concept abduction: these are possibilities, a 'state' of experience in the absolute present, which are basic singular qualities that may combine in various ways to introduce novel things into the world. Once conceived, they are introduced into the universe of ideas that might be considered for a new category of inquiry to be subjected to the processes of scientific induction and deduction.

Maslow's account of human behavior focuses on human motivation based on people seeking fulfillment and change through personal growth doing all they are capable of achieving. Maslow's account focuses on what goes right not on what goes wrong. He stated that a person finds meaning in life that is important to them. Motivation for self-actualization leads people differently: creating works of art, literature, sport, classroom, or corporate success. Maslow's categories are useful to guide engineers in developing an artifact, but the idea ascending levels of human need is problematic.

Consider Victor Frankl's premise that humans are motivated by a "will to meaning," an inner pull to find meaning in life whatever their current level of need. Value = Artifact (for an Engineer) which
- Is derived in engineering design between developer, marketing and customer.
- Satisfies Cost Benefit Analysis for an organization constrained by value for a sustainable society.
- Improves socioeconomic criteria measured by Net Present Value, Balanced Score Card, GDP.
- Considers Frankl's will to meaning.

Since artifacts created by engineers within the socio-cultural system have been a major contributor to the crisis of social harm from digital platforms, engineers must be engaged in all aspects of the solution including defining the problem, developing the requirements, and proposing solutions within a strategy and portfolio of programs and projects.

III Engineering Philosophy

A philosophy of engineering is made up of:
- Epistemology: A theory of knowledge
- Ontology: A theory of being
- Axiology: A theory of value

This paper presents Engineering concepts based on KNOWLEDGE (epistemology) FLOW (ontology) TO VALUE (axiology) , defining elements of engineering and societal communities and finally describing an expanded view of value within an ethical engineering process which establishes how:
- An engineer's observation leads to the leaps of faith required for implementing tangible improvement from novelty.
- A design engineering team validates novelty and delivers a prototype to validate a design.
- A production engineering team validates a prototype and constructs capability to deliver it in quantity with quality.

The current crises are related to how social media is creating harmful effects across all of society and all of the political, economic, social and technological institutions.

Habermas perspective is particularly useful in understanding why this has occurred. Further philosophical foundations, and a philosophy of engineering, are needed to understand how this might be mitigated and fixed.

An Engineering Philosophy that can solve for the current crises must embrace a code of ethics necessary to guide society to a universal value system, which could be embedded into digital platforms. The current conflicts and societal harms might in fact be the result of the tensions between the multitude of value systems represented by the evolving destructive, tribal nature of internet communities.

This section presents some element of a general philosophy of engineering and its application to the current crises with digital platforms.

Human life, institutions and all disciplines are driven by existing value systems which engineering embraces. Many people believe in a god and engineering purports to deliver value to humanity; philosophy must embrace a concept of a god (or higher power) that acts as a necessary (but not necessarily sufficient) condition to get us beyond Heidegger's enframing and to systems of institutions and platforms that support the health, wealth and well-being of people, in otherwards higher order values.

The engineering challenge to fix the harmful aspects of digital platforms, and then improve them, requires additional philosophical perspectives related to novelty and novel solutions, innovation, process, consciousness, reliability, cognition and creativity.

The following additional perspectives provide more foundation for an engineering philosophy that forms the basis of some governing principles for managing the current crises.

Novelty defines, for example, the innovative features of digital platforms. Novelty can be revealed as an extrapolation of mathematics or scientific theory but, most new knowledge and therefore innovations are revealed by intuition – seeing things in ways never observed before. Newton's Laws, Darwin's Theory, Confucius' analects, Christ's parables, art, literature, engineering, mathematics, architecture, technology, and science are evidence of a continuous stream of novelty from revelation. All explicitly defined knowledge either comes from an individual's mind or is revealed to an individual's mind.

In his Theory of Organism, Whitehead proposes that the only reality is process, that everything has a form of intelligence and that objects change moment to moment . We each see projections of reality, considerably altered by one's fields of consciousness. The question to be answered is: how does one transcend a limited perception of reality to acquire new insights? Whitehead proposes reality is a dynamic stream of consciousness. Social platforms connect us in ways that often change how we perceive reality before we are ready for it. In this case the process of engaging with an engineered artifact (platform) is as important as the artifact itself.

Kuhn's paradigms describe how engineers communicate effectively and also provide the foundation for explaining how engineering radically changes when viable novel ideas are introduced and validated.

Beer's VSM and Pyzdek's Six Sigma methodologies define in detail how to model and change any business, societal, government or ecological environment using a PMI portfolio of programs and projects.

Descartes' Subject/Object Metaphysics (SOM) assumed our human senses are the only reality we can rely on. Whitehead thinks otherwise. Whitehead provides a detailed view of how one's mind processes external stimuli as constituted in the past (causal efficacy), as taken up into the present (presentational immediacy) and as reference to immediate future (symbolic reference). Since the two primitive modes of perception are incapable of error, symbolic reference (human conscious) introduces this possibility.

Viewing digital platforms through this lens is useful for understanding how they affect us moment to moment and their impact on our perceptions of reality and why platforms have been so good at changing behavior. Whitehead's ultimate principle of reality is a process event called an occasion. Creativity does not exist in any other form than occasions. Whitehead says that creativity is novelty of instance. Novelty of instance is a new result derived from previously actualized old data; novelty of kind introduces new data into the stream of process.

Social platforms introduce new concepts so rapidly that they change our perceptions dynamically and quickly, and our behaviours may change subconsciously by how we feel before our rational, conscious minds can catch up. Fast changing perceptions make individual reality very dynamic and this has become one real effect of relationships on social platforms.

Finally, Kant's *Formula of Humanity* is considered to be the most intuitively appealing formulation of the imperative to treat persons with dignity and respect, we must always treat each other as ends in themselves and never as mere means . This suggests an approach to how we should manage the ways the maturity of our cultures are deteriorating, mostly due to social harms from digital platforms.

Throughout the rich and developed world, we are not living through a crisis of wealth or material, but a crisis of character, a crisis of virtue, a crisis of means and ends. The fundamental political schism in 2024 is no longer right versus left, but the compromised values of both the right and left. It's no longer a debate of socialism versus capitalism or freedom versus equity but, rather, of power and electability, of the immaturity of a global collective social intelligence and of means versus ends.

IV Knowledge Flow to Value

Having looked at elements of engineering philosophy this section presents key concepts about knowledge and value that need to be equally understood. Here we introduce knowledge management and types of knowledge in order to bring a pragmatic perspective into the philosophy of engineering. We also introduce system engineering methodology to describe how engineers communicate.

Every useful act can be viewed as, knowledge flow (from noise) to value.
- Noise -> Data -> Information -> knowledge (tacit, skills, prescriptive)
- Value = Artifact (for an Engineer)
- Flow represents an organization's processes.

	Wisdom	
	Understanding	
	Knowledge	
Information & Observations		
Facts & Data		
Noise & Nonsense & Novelty		

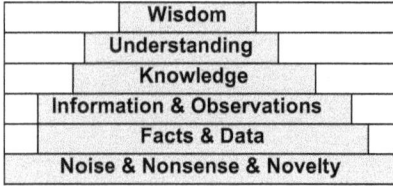

Fig. 1 Knowledge Hierarchy

Knowledge validates information. Here are standard knowledge definitions from Knowledge management in Figure 1 which over-simplistically derive one from another.

- Noise is any undifferentiated thing assaulting the senses; it is pervasive, ubiquitous, auditory, visual, textural.
- Data is derived noise when it transcends the purely sensual and has cognitive pattern; when it can be discerned and differentiated by the mind (this transition of noise to data is nonsense: it is much more involved to differentiate reality from noise).
- Information is derived from data when it is assembled into a coherent whole which can be related to other information in a way that adds meaning . . . a difference that makes a difference.
- Knowledge is derived from verified, validated information when it has interacted with other information in a form useful for deciding, acting, or composing new validated knowledge.
- Understanding is derived from knowledge when related to other knowledge in a manner useful in conceiving, anticipating, evaluating, and judging.
- Wisdom comes from understanding when informed by purpose, ethics, principle, memory of the past and projection into the future.

Knowledge Management implies data is derived from noise easily. It is not. Noise comes in a variety of forms:
- data recorded with uncalibrated instruments
- false statements and theories
- unsubstantiated claims to be scientific or knowledge
- irrelevant statements about a person's activities
- observations derived from bad data
- information that incorrectly summarizes data
- information derived from an inadequate data
- large volumes of irrelevant data (AI, Big Data)
- conclusions from cherry picked facts
- conclusion drawn from out-of-context knowledge
- knowledge imbedded in a cloud of nonsense
- assertions falsely claiming scientific derivation
- claims of causation from correlation in data
- hypothesis posing as (untested) theories
- corrupt data, information, knowledge anomalies.

Extracting data, information, and knowledge from Internet noise and real life can be an extensive time-consuming process. But there may be novelty in the noise that could precipitate a new reality.

Knowledge includes tacit, skills, empirical, prescriptive, and scientific knowledge constrained by maintainability and sustainability. These categories are centered on learning various processes to acquire knowledge in engineering and technology.

Tacit Knowledge cannot be explained or justified; it has an important role in many forms of craftsmanship. For instance, drywallers can seldom explain the hand movements by which they even out a surface much faster, and with much less spackling, than an amateur. Three different purposes in engineering require the need to articulate tacit knowledge:
- Facilitating the mechanization of a work process previously performed by craftspeople.
- Facilitating teaching and learning. Articulation makes learning possible without long apprenticeships.
- Controlling other people's work by systematically codifying the extensive (tacit and explicit) knowledge of experienced workers into subtasks that can easily be taught, learned, and performed by less qualified labor or partially automated by AI and other systems.

Practical Rule Knowledge: Developed by trial and error as "rule-of-thumb" such as making load-bearing parts strong enough to carry twice the intended load but has no theory to choose '2' as a safety factor. With rule-of-thumb knowledge, it is often advantageous to routinize it making it possible to perform a task with at most sporadic attention. For example, an experienced truck driver shifts gears up or down without thinking.

Systematic Engineering Knowledge is obtained through studies by engineering scientists in universities and industry. Through the centuries, technological development has been driven by craftsmen systematically trying out different constructions and methods. E.g., new metallurgic methods are based on experience.

Applied Natural Science: Engineers were educated in mathematics and physics late in the 19th century to employ natural science to develop new technology. Since then, knowledge came from many areas: physics, chemistry, biology, and earth sciences. Technology is now also based on natural science, tacit and rule knowledge, and knowledge based on systematic investigations of technological constructions.

Idealization in Engineering Science means to restrict one's attention to certain important properties to study an object and not get lost in detail. Idealization may involve a distortion of the original or it can mean leaving aside some components in a complex object to better focus on the remaining ones.

Engineering science has important metaphysical and epistemological differences from natural science:

- It serves the needs of a profession, namely engineers.
- Its objects of study are human made, not natural objects.
- Its objects must be understood in terms of complex combinations of physical and functional characteristics.
- Its epistemology incorporates forms of systematized action-guiding knowledge not based on natural science.
- It operates on a less abstract level than the natural sciences, and refrains from many of their idealizations.
- Novelty is something incomprehensively new requiring theory, validation, and subsequent generalization into one or more forms of engineering knowledge.

V Systems Engineering

In this section we add methodology to further ground the practical nature of the philosophy of engineering. Value of an object or service has many different aspects (see Table I).

Table I. Aspects to Consider in Artifact Design

Quality	Whitehead's Process & Reality NASA Systems Engineering Guide . Standards: ISO 9001 / ISO15489 / 6 Sigma
Ethics Morality	IEEE Code of Conduct, Hippocratic Oath, etc… Seven Virtues, Seven Sins, Mores, Duty, Rules Theology – Christianity; Islam; Judaism; Hinduism; Daoism; Panentheism
Economy /Industry	NPV, ROI, BSC, CBA in 19 Sectors: Manufacturing, Healthcare, Energy, Aerospace, Agriculture, Computer, Telecommunication, Education, Construction, Electronics, Mining, Transport, Pharmaceutical, Entertainment, World Wide Web, News, Media, Music, Food, Hospitality
Health	Medicare for all with co-pays based on age Michael Porter's IPU for Healthcare Delivery ,
Social Science	Utopia: Plato, Jesus, Thomas More, John Rawls Law: (no dystopia): Hobbes (Leviathan), Montesquieu (USA), Locke, Smith, Rousseau Model (Habermas) WEF GCI
Ecological Science	WEF GCI with IoT and sustainability criteria Energy – Dual fuel hybrid vehicles, EVs, NG pipelines, Constrained Fracking Local Solar, Wind/Hydro/Upgraded Nuclear power Habitat – GMO fertilizer/pesticides/crops (increase yield/soil restoration) Lumbering - strip cut not clear-cut forests

Maslow Human Needs	1. Biological and physiological: air, food, drink, shelter, warmth, sex, sleep, etc.
	2. Safety: protection from elements, security, order, law, stability, etc.
	3. Love & belonging: friendship, intimacy, trust, acceptance: family, friends, work.
	4. Esteem: dignity, achievement, mastery, independence; respect (status, prestige).
	5. Cognitive: understanding, curiosity, exploration, need for meaning and predictability.
	6. Aesthetic: appreciation and search for beauty, balance, form, etc.
	7. Self-actualization: realizing personal potential, self-fulfilment, seeking personal growth.
	8. Transcendence: beyond the self (mysticism, nature, service, pursuit of science, religion, etc.).

The underlying system engineering methodology presented here assumes that for an organization to be even viable, it must deliver/process 'value' of some sort. This section will postulate the types of value that may make an artifact (product or service) appeal to people.

Value is usually guided less by ethics and intellectual pursuits than it is by profit, utility, recreation, comfort, and security. And while engineering transforms humankind by leveraging knowledge to create new and novel artifacts. Engineering must evolve to provide a system and discipline that is moral and sustainable to:
1] Benefit Individual well-being,
2] Precipitate and validate Novelty,
3] Charge societies with sustainable value,
4] Provide foundation to create high-value artifacts,

Engineers gain significant insights from knowledge flow to value but may opt not to commission an initial model to identify elements of an environment or because they would prefer to focus on explicitly solvable rather than a complex adaptive problem. Organizational and government bureaucrats have had no model of knowledge flow to value to set policy, so proposed solutions frequently inflict more harm than good. Bureaucrats must know how knowledge flows to value to set policy and outline a portfolio on how to better leverage existing skills, processes, and technology with a change methodology like Six Sigma to improve a local process with the assurance that it improves organization's artifact delivery process.

VI Knowledge flow to value in Firms

To grasp how these philosophies help us to understand, govern and manage digital platforms and any other engineered artifact, it is important to further grasp knowledge flow to value in institutions. Knowledge Flow to Value can represent all businesses, organizations, institutions, entities, engineering and systems engineering.

Understanding, quantifying, and optimizing knowledge flow to value is defined in philosophical terms enumerated in Table II.

A clear philosophical position enriches and frames the methodology that is applied to engineer a new artifact, a new feature or new benefit (on a platform, for example). This method is based on an assembly of robust methodologies guided by economic, ethical, aesthetic, and sustainable valuations.

Table II. Philosophy Definitions

Episte-mology Know-ledge	Theory of knowledge: the study of the nature, origin and scope of human knowledge and cognition, its justification and rationality of belief, and issues related to its use.
Ontology / Meta-physics Flow	Theory of reality: the study of being in general, or of what applies neutrally to everything that is real. Modern use of ontology is a way to show the properties of a subject area and how they are related, by defining a set of concepts and categories to represent a framework for the subject area.
Axiology Value	Theory of value: the study of goodness, or value. Its significance lies in the expansion given to the meaning of value to provide for the study of a variety of questions: economic, aesthetic, ethic, and sustainability in delivery of artifacts—usually considered in relative isolation.
Artifact	Objects or services for human beings based on: • Economics: ROI, CBA, time-to-market… • Ethics: standards or codes of behavior appropriate in certain social groups. • Aesthetics: art, taste, and beauty (from an object's property or a feeling it provokes). • Sustainability: maintenance, restoration, and ecological, political, and social sciences. • Social: impacts on social groups and society. • Political: impact on professions and governments.

Engineering as we know it in the 21st century has many specialist disciplines: E.g., Electrical, Aerospace, Computer, Chemical, Biomedical, Environmental, Civil, Mechanical, and Systems Engineering. Table III lists the disciplines from Professional Engineers Book of Knowledge.

Table III. Engineering Book of Knowledge

Capability	Professional Engineering Body of Knowledge		
Basic	Mathematics	Natural sciences	Humanities
Technical	Manufacturing	Design	Economics
	Science	Tools	Problem solving
	Quality control	Risk /reliability	Safety
	Societal impact	Systems	Maintenance
	Sustainability	Technical breadth	Technical depth
Professional Practice	Business	Communication	Ethics
	Global awareness	Leadership	Legal
	Teamwork	Learning	Profession
	Project Mgt	Public policy	

System Engineering Methodology describes how engineers must communicate across these specialist disciplines and within groups to successfully design, develop, validate, prototype, and redesign for manufacture, management, and delivery of artifacts for human use and consumption. It must consider demands made by consumers, management, quality, cost, development, materials, manufacturability, maintainability, and the engineering community standards, codes of ethics, and constraints.

The paper's focus is on Systems Engineering because it represents the ways in which engineering projects are managed within and between other engineering disciplines, mechanical, electrical and information.

VII Philosophy of Engineering

This paper defines a Philosophy of Engineering based on the principles outlined above: To reiterate, KNOWLEDGE (epistemology) FLOW (ontology) TO VALUE (axiology) based on how:

• An engineer's transcendent observation leads to design novelty (revelation).
• A design engineering team validates revelation and delivers a protype to validate the design.
• A production engineering team validates the prototype and constructs a capability to deliver it.

Value is represented by an artifact which can be an object or service that someone uses for a benefit. The artifact can be medical interventions, automobiles, phones, legal counselling, software features etc. To create a sustainable environment is dependent upon the ability to explicitly define, monitor and continuously improve knowledge flow-to-value for features in products, services, delivery, and restoration.

A document (page, news feed, etc), for example may contain noise, data, information, or knowledge, even misinformation and fake information. Noise is an incomprehensible jumble of images, sounds, and text. Data can result from monitoring events or is derived from other data. Information is the result of summarizing or correlating data; it is data organized into patterns and visualized to create insights that support decisions. Knowledge is actionable information because it has meaning; it has been validated from collaboration, and quality of method; analytical, statistical, and logical methods are used to build an information base that is reviewed by a peer group to validate structure and content.

Figure 1 earlier illustrates transition from noise to knowledge. Value in an organization is primarily driven by competition where customers know the value of products. KNOWLEDGE FLOW TO VALUE represents a system engineering method for knowledge flow to value consulting.

The transition from noise to knowledge can change attitudes and behavior as evidenced by many organizational digital transformation projects in the past few decades.

However, changing part of an organization and expecting the entire organization to improve is problematic and often unreasonable. Many change initiatives fail at great cost, some cause negative, unintended consequences. One basic reason underlies this failure: the knowledge to manage and change the organization was not well understood or it was ignored. Several of the many knowledge-related business problems include:

- When people leave an organization, unless knowledge in their heads and skills has been captured and transferred to those remaining or is explicitly documented, a valuable asset is lost.
- Hoarding occurs when the cultural theme is "knowledge is power," it does not flow crippling organizations.
- Unsubstantiated assertions pose as facts; testing and validation are required for information to be considered knowledge. A clear distinction must be made between claims and verified knowledge.
- Knowledge shelf-life: there are "time-honored truths" and "yesterday's news." The challenge is assuring a given 'packet' of knowledge persists through an extended life cycle and knowing when to discard it.
- Intangible knowledge is difficult to manage directly.

An organization must manage the entire knowledge environment to accelerate knowledge flow to deliver quality artifacts. A method must enable an enterprise to capture critical knowledge and connect it to those who need it. To manage knowledge within an enterprise includes defining a body of knowledge comprising instructions, skills, theories, rules, processes, techniques for action used by a firm to solve problems and produce artifacts; explicit knowledge is recorded in documents; unrecorded knowledge is discovered by:

- analyzing the entire body of knowledge to identify a plurality of knowledge objects which itemize and encapsulates specific knowledge that is used by enterprise processes to produce outputs having value;
- defining a measurable process environment comprising measurable enterprise processes, wherein the processes use the identified knowledge objects to produce artifacts having value;
- assembling a taxonomy for the enterprise comprising a system for classifying the knowledge objects; and classifying all recorded and unrecorded knowledge objects according to the taxonomy.
- measuring the flow of each knowledge object through its monitored process to produce the output to determine a measured baseline flow for the knowledge object;
- modifying processes from measured flow until optimized flow for its knowledge objects have

been achieved while capturing all recorded and unrecorded knowledge object flow in documents.

The method further includes periodically redefining the body of knowledge to solve problems and produce better artifacts faster. Note that *documents* are the containers for all forms of explicit knowledge.

The System Engineering Methodology described here is based on the author's Document Methodology that asserts documents record enterprise and institutional knowledge, define process, provide facts to manage people, structure support systems, and guide change and engineering.

VIII Professions, Communities, Models

When a system is correctly designed, a human user can employ it in a deliberate manner to deliver the desired outcomes at the desired time. At this abstract level, technical systems can be described through a black box that shows inputs and outputs.

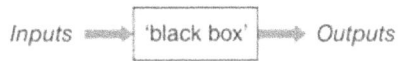

Inputs ══► ¦'black box'¦ ══► Outputs

Fig. 2 Black box causally links an input to a (desired) output

This black box (figure 2) approach has been used to manifest the first abstract representation of systems to be designed, managed and governed. The representation is then broken down into inherent actions or technical processes that transform the given inputs until they reach the final output states. Combining all relevant operational functions into a causal, logical chain, in which the output of one serves as input for the next, establishes the comprehensive functional structure of a system.

This structure then serves as a coherent representation of the inherent mechanisms, processes, transformations, and their relations of how the system functions, i.e. how it operates, to establish the causal relation between inputs and outputs and how people engage with the system to derive benefit. All these internal operations thus comprise the system's functionality. As such the abstract concept describes the distinct actions and effectual causes, and their relations, taking place in a system to achieve a desired outcome.

An artifact is an object deliberately made in a system for a human being. It can take the form of a product, digital system, service, or any assembly thereof. It is part of every design process; artifacts have a dual nature. On the one hand, an artifact is a physical object or service that can be used to accomplish a specific goal; on the other, it is an intentional object or service, whose function has meaning within the context of a broader set of goal-oriented human activities. Artifacts function and intentionality create this dual nature between physical and/or process structure and perceived value (Figure 3).

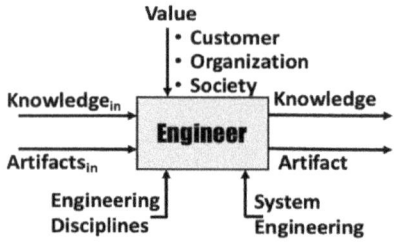

Fig. 3 Engineer links an input to a desired artifact

Communities are populated by individuals who have acquired and used knowledge and skills to support critical areas of society and also serve to critique the novel ideas of its members. Scientific theories are validated in communities by experiments, predicted observations, and/or confirmation of mathematical derivations. In a scientific or engineering community theories are viewed skeptically, especially if it invalidates established theories. The Physics community ostracized Albert Einstein until his Theory of Relativity was validated by observation of cosmological phenomenon. Engineering theory is easier to validate; it works for a specific category of problems, or it doesn't.

Communities have supported critical areas of society. What is their purpose? What are the criteria for membership into the various communities? How do they operate? What purpose should it serve?

Engineering societies resemble craftsmen's guilds. To become a junior engineer, one must first be educated in a university with an accredited engineering program. However, having the knowledge acquired at such an institution is not enough. All engineers subscribe to the adage: if you build it, it must work. Many apprentice engineers work for a corporation where they become part of a guild-like engineering community. Apprentice engineers learn how to design, validate and build things that work.

A scientific theory and engineering method is usually felt to be better than its predecessors if it is a better instrument for discovering and solving puzzles.

A way to coordinate engineering among different disciplines being used within a project is a Community of Practice (CoP) where disparate engineering teams can share information, insight, experience, and tools about an area specific to their project. They facilitate internal and external communication to determine best practices and transfer organizational knowledge within and across divisions and disciplines.

Engineering Professional Code of ethics applies only to voluntary participants in a special practice, not to everyone; a code (if followed) can create trust beyond what ordinary moral conduct can by creating a special ethical environment. For example, a code of ethics can justify trust in the claims of an engineer beyond the trust those claims would deserve if the engineer were just an ordinary decent person.

Professions are designed to serve a certain moral ideal, that is, to contribute to a state of affairs everyone can recognize as good to achieve. So, physicians have organized to cure the sick, comfort the dying, and protect the healthy from disease; lawyers, to help people obtain justice within the law; engineers, to improve the material condition of humanity.

A profession does not just organize to serve a certain moral ideal; it organizes to serve it in a certain way, that is, according to standards beyond what law, market, morality, and public opinion would otherwise require. IEEE's code of ethics (not listed here) is an outstanding example which has three other legitimate uses:

1] help "the public" understand what may be expected of any engineer and what engineers expect of themselves.

2] provide a vocabulary to interpret technical standards, e.g., "your specification, puts public safety at risk."

3] help engineers resist pressure from client, or superior to do what they should n

Systems engineering is common across all engineering disciplines and manages the progress of one or more of these disciplines to create an artifact (e.g., iPhone, car, plane, etc.).

Communication technology and engineering are precipitating innovations at a rapid rate in the public sphere precipitating Habermas' legitimation crisis in all three systems. Since people's lives are value driven, system engineering must embrace and resolve this crisis in a changing world.

Models are used to show the interrelationships between all of the functions of a system. Figure 4 represents interactions of a network of four high-level models that regulate, manage and support an enterprise or an institution:

• **Government** regulates the market within which the enterprise operates.

• **Manage** is a recursive view of management that directs all levels of the business.

- **Support** represents the support systems that drive knowledge flow to value.

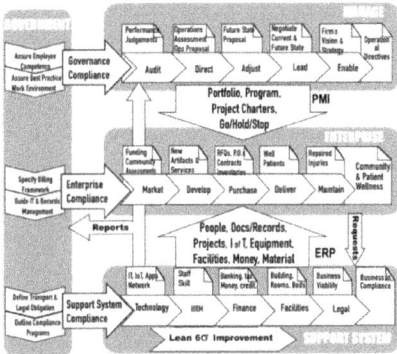

Figure 4 Enterprise Model Network

- **Enterprise** is the high-level process of the firm. The core upper-level enterprise functions are:
  - Market: educate customers with timely, accurate proposals.
  - Develop: create desirable, sustainable artifacts defined by design documents.
  - Purchase: acquire resources from trusted, reliable suppliers using documents to facilitate transactions.
  - Deliver: provide quality, low-cost artifacts delivered on-time, guided by transaction documents.
  - Maintain: ensure satisfied customers using maintenance, scheduling, & account history documents.

Note: "Audit" within the manage process evaluates the statistics and information generated from the operation of enterprise. This type of audit can also be applied to the operation of government and to the operations of digital AI platforms.

Legitimation crisis in political, cultural, and economic systems have resulted in citizens losing confidence in society: both at international and national levels, social platforms are making this worse in many instances. Institutional structures need continuously engineered innovation (novelty), to assure sustainability and benefits. Auditing government performance and misbehavior will require a special audit that first extracts statistics and information from Internet misinformation and propaganda. The value that is derived from this audit can be government and business transparency which concerned citizens can use to determine who should govern them (if they care).

Up until now, people with biases have judged the accuracy of an assertion; AI used in the contexts described here may be a better impartial arbiter. AI won't find the truth, but we would expect it to help identify disparities in information and its

sources. Humans must draw conclusions. AI can identify disparities in an audit and suggest solutions to disparities.

In this case AI is used to help manage complexity. But AI is not reliable without an added context of collaboration amongst people. This is necessary because individuals cannot cope in isolation with complexity. Therefore organizations foster collaboration to form autonomous units, accountable for chunks of complexity; these are the organization's primary activities. Each autonomous unit is functionally specialized in producing an aspect of the organization's purposes.

Candidates to perform this audit could include the processes and systems used in ship classification societies which are non-governmental organizations that establish and maintain technical standards for the construction and operation of ships and offshore structures. Some societies have expanded their audit to other industries.

Det Norske Veritas group (DNV), the largest of these organizations, has expanded its auditing beyond maritime to include power, oil and gas, automotive and aerospace, food and beverage, healthcare, and other industries. In *Assurance of AI-Enabled Systems* the DNV sets out a comprehensive process for auditing AI and could be extended to social platforms to mitigate the current crises of societal harm, misinformation and disinformation from digital AI platforms. The DNV practice is to create a framework for assuring AI-enabled systems, which we contend can be extended to digital platforms. It includes:
- methodological details that support the assurance process.
- how to strengthen the knowledge about system properties and outputs, and thereby provide confidence that the system meets expectations.
- a method for case-specific system requirements for assuring warranted trust in the capabilities of systems and for managing AI and platforms responsibly.
- how to show compliance with the case-specific requirements and applicable standards throughout the lifecycle.

This recommended practice does not cover the assurance of organizations involved in AI-enabled systems and digital platforms, such as an institutions' management systems or work process. These were covered elsewhere in this paper.

Further guided by the engineering philosophy outlined here, the DNV is an example of a set of practices that could be a candidate for establishing a capability for an agile independent body as a key element to regulation, standards and standard processes necessary to address risks and ensure we can trust information and platforms we are using.

This is an essential step to trusting digital platforms, AI, and the institutions and people that use these technologies. Scaling this to a global capability should essentially give us an ability to trust our political institutions, better identify with our economic institutions, committing to social institutions while learning to keep our technological institutions viable, creating a better future as a collective for everyone.

IX Summary and Conclusions
This paper raises concerns about the misuse of AI and digital platforms, highlighting the spread of harmful content and risks posed by technologically advanced artifacts. It points to the urgent need for a multi-stakeholder collaboration to establish ethical foundations and governance practices for technology. The role of engineers is emphasized as central to addressing these challenges, advocating for an engineering philosophy that prioritizes ethics and sustainable value creation.

The ideas and methods presented here, including the philosophies and philosophers mentioned, provide the foundation for understanding how engineers ideate and think, communicate, and work in groups to design, develop, validate, prototype, redesign, manage themselves, and manufacture artifacts. They must consider consumers, management, quality, cost, material, availability, development, manufacture, maintenance, standards, codes of ethics, and societal constraints.

A Philosophy of Engineering based on Knowledge Flow to Value and network of models that represent institutions embedded in society and audited by an independent body provides a foundation for regulating, guiding regulators, and auditing both.

A Philosophy of Engineering based on **Knowledge Flow to Value** establishes how (via Peirce):
- An engineer's transcendent observation leads to design novelty (Abduction).
- A design engineering team validates revelation and delivers a protype to validate the design (Deduction).
- A production engineering team validates the prototype and constructs a capability to deliver it (Induction).

The paper underscores the importance of broad discourse and a systematic approach to engineering, suggesting that such strategies are vital for mitigating the negative impacts of AI and ensuring the responsible use of technology.

X References
- American Productivity & Quality Centre, Process Classification Framework
- Beer, Stafford, The Heart of Enterprise, Wiley & Sons Ltd, 1979
- DNV, RECOMMENDED PRACTICE, DNV-RP-067, Assurance of AI-enabled Systems, 2023
- Frankl, Viktor E., Man's Search for Meaning, Beacon Press, 1959
- Habermas, Juergen, Moral Consciousness and Communicative Action, MIT Press, 1990
- Heidegger, Martin, Being and Time, Harper Row, 1962
- Jones, Jeffrey I., Collective Social Intelligence, Austin Macauley Publisher, Ltd. London, 2017
- Jones, Jim I. and Jones, Jeffrey I., Ethics and Knowledge in Engineering, IEEE, 2022
- Jones, Jim I. and Jones, Jeffrey I., Optimizing Healthcare, IEEE HEALTHCOM, Szechuan, China, Mar 2021
- Jones, Jim I., The Document Methodology, 1999, Version II 2007, Version III 2019.
- Jones, Jim I., US Patent Application 20040102990: Method to Manage Knowledge Flow to Value, 2003
- Kant, Immanuel, Metaphysics of Morals, Categorical Imperative, 1780
- Kuhn, Thomas S., The Structure of Scientific Revolutions, University of Chicago Press, 1962
- Mcleod, Saul, Maslow's Hierarchy of Needs, simplypsychology.org/maslow.html, 2007, 2022
- NASA, Systems Engineering Handbook, 2007
- National Society of Professional Engineers, PE Body of Knowledge, 2013
- Peirce, John Sanders and Buchler, Justus, Philosophical Writings of Peirce, Dover Publications, March 2011
- Porter, Michael E. and Teisberg, Elizabeth O., Redefining Healthcare, HBS Press, 2006.
- Project Management Institute, Portfolio, Program and Project Management Standards
- Pyzdek, Thomas, The Six Sigma Handbook Version IV, McGraw Hill, 2014
- Seidel, Jamie, How a 'confused' AI may have fought pilots attempting to save Boeing 737 MAX8s,19Mar2019
- Stanford Encyclopedia of Philosophy, 2021
- Warren, Todd, wardsauto.com/industry-news/software-related-recalls-and-auto-industry-s-ongoing-evolution, 24Feb2024
- WEF GCI Report, www.weforum.org /reports/the-global-competitveness-report-2018.
- WEF Global Risks Report 2024, www.weforum.org/ publications/global-risks-report-2024/
- Whitehead, A. N., Process and Reality, 1929
- Whitehead, A. N., Religion in the Making, 1926
- Zuboff, Shoshana, The Age of Surveillance Capitalism, Profile, 2019

Author: Dr. Jim I. Jones

Dr. Jones is a Systems Engineer with experience in the U.S., Germany, England, and Australia in management, development and consulting positions in information systems, CAD/CAM/CIM and systems engineering. He has provided information management and planning consulting services to companies such as Newcrest Mining, Ericsson, Siemens, Ford, Compaq, Xerox, Lear Seating, Deere & Co., Lockheed - Martin, General Motors, Adam Opel, and TCI.

Dr. Jones has been employed in the U.S. and Europe in a variety of development, consulting, and management positions in information systems and engineering for 23 years at General Motors. In his nine years at CIMLINC, a software technology company, he was Vice President of Development and Vice President of Product Marketing.

Acknowledgements

This methodology embraces concepts of many excellent scholars, and it is built on the experience that has solved problems in disparate industries. By allowing me to solve a variety of problems, Xerox, Lockheed-Martin, Ford, Deere & Co, TCI, Gambro Healthcare, Ericsson, Siemens, CIMLINC, GM and Newcrest Mining have contributed to developing The Document Methodology. Authors who had a significant role in TDM include Stafford Beer, W. Edwards Deming, Eli Goldratt, Alan Pritsker and Michael Porter.

Doug Foran, Bob Haglund, Jim Hogan, Jeff and John Jones, Jim MacDonald, A.J. Meyer, Ken Morrison, Alan Pritsker, Ted Powers, Lothar Rossol, Adrian Sannier, Jim Spillman, Cornelia Stinchcomb, Tom Starr and Charles White critiqued Version I. Mohamed Arif, Cliff Bamford, David Dirks, Doug Foran, Dennis Kulonda, David Mills, and Mike Sterling critiqued Version II. Jeff Jones, Dennis Kulonda, Kristina Reynolds, Mike Sterling and Judith A. Ryan critiqued Version III.

Again, I owe a special thanks to Judith G. Jones (BA, RN, WIFE) for her invaluable contributions to all four editions of this work.

www.ingramcontent.com/pod-product-compliance
Lightning Source LLC
Chambersburg PA
CBHW040901210326
41597CB00029B/4927